hand reflexology

simple routines for health and relaxation

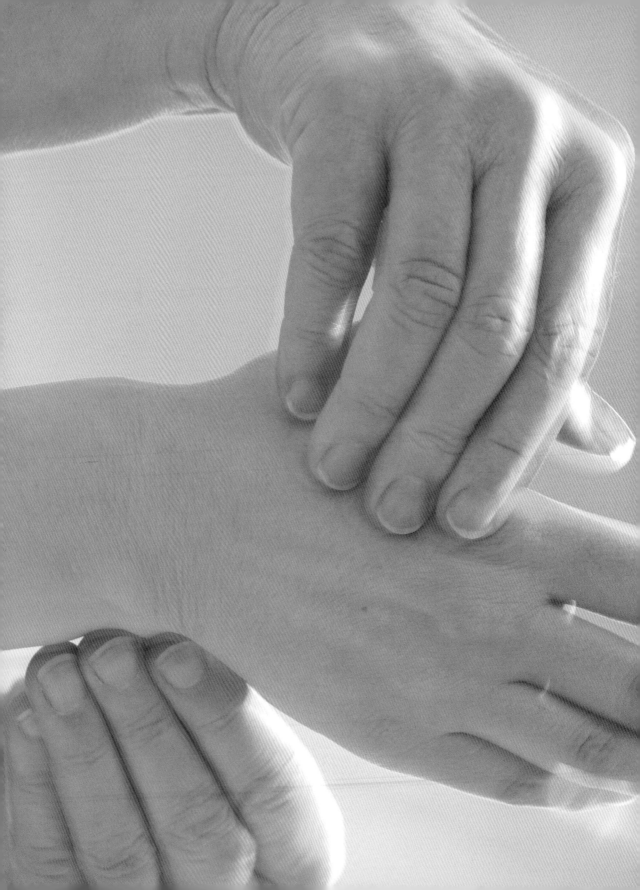

hand reflexology

simple routines for health and relaxation

BARBARA & KEVIN KUNZ

PHOTOGRAPHY BY
RUTH JENKINSON

LONDON, NEW YORK, MELBOURNE,
MUNICH, and DELHI

Editor: Irene Lyford
Art Editor: Toni Kay
Senior Editor: Shannon Beatty
Senior Art Editor: Peggy Sadler
Managing Editor: Penny Warren
Managing Art Editor: Marianne Markham
Publishing Operations Manager: Gillian Roberts
Creative Publisher: Mary-Clare Jerram
Art Director: Peter Luff
Publishing Director: Corinne Roberts
DTP Designer: Sonia Charbonnier
Production Controller: Maria Elia

First American Edition 2006
06 07 08 09 10 9 8 7 6 5 4 3

Published in the United States by DK Publishing
375 Hudson Street, New York, New York 10014

DK books are available at special discounts for bulk
purchases for sales promotions, premiums, fund-raising,
or educational use. For details contact DK Publishing
Special Markets, 375 Hudson Street, New York,
NY 10014 or SpecialSales@dk.com

Cataloging-in-Publication data is available from
the Library of Congress
ISBN-10: 0-7566-2060-0
ISBN-13: 978-0-7566-2060-8

Color reproduction by Colourscan, Singapore
Printed and bound in China by Sheck Wah Tong
Discover more at **www.dk.com**

CONTENTS

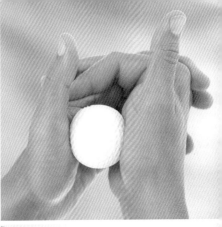

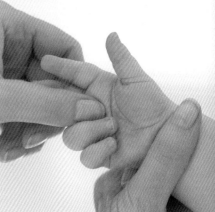

6 Introduction

8 Principles of reflexology

The history of reflexology 10 • How reflexology works 12
Reflexology and zones 14 • Hand reflexology maps 16

20 Benefits of reflexology

Why do people use hand reflexology? 22 • Advantages
of hand reflexology 24 • Reflexology for everyone 26
Reflexology research 29 • Reflexology in medical care 30
Success stories 32 • Visiting a reflexologist 34

36 Taking care of your hands

Anatomy of the hand 38 • Ergonomics and the hands 40
Hands: an owner's manual 42 • Using self-help tools 44
Relaxation exercises 46

48 The hand-reflexology session

Preparing for a reflexology session 50 • Techniques 54
Hand desserts 60 • The complete hand-reflexology
sequence 66 • Self-help hand desserts 82 • The complete
self-help hand-reflexology sequence 86 • The complete golf-
ball self-help hand-reflexology sequence 102 • People with
specific needs 110 • Reflexology at the office 114
Reflexology on the move 116 • Reflexology on the road 118

120 Reflexology to target health concerns

Using reflexology for health concerns 122 • Stress 124
Headaches 126 • Backache & neck pain 128 • Pain 130
Breast cancer recovery 132 • Other health concerns 134
Using reflexology for hand concerns 140 • Keyboarding
142 • Sporting hands 144 • Tired & sore hands 146 • Carpal
tunnel syndrome 148 • Arthritis 150 • Hand injury 152

154 Finding a reflexologist • Contacts
155 Websites and further reading
156 Index
160 Acknowledgments

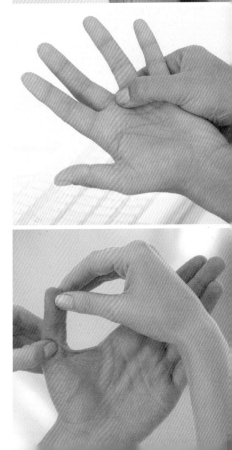

INTRODUCTION

Hands occupy a very special place in our lives: every day, tIme and time again, we call upon them to perform tasks that range from the mundane to the intricate, from a gentle caress to exerting extreme force. Because of their special relationship with the body, the hands provide a unique opportunity for addressing health concerns. Hand reflexology seizes the chance of enhancing not only your own life but also that of others. Its techniques can provide busy hands with a respite from the demands of the day; but, more importantly, reflexology can change lives. From the worker whose livelihood is threatened by disability to the senior citizen seeking to live independently, hand reflexology offers possibilities of improvement and offers a path to pursue in times of need.

This point was driven home to us a number of years ago during a demonstration at a rehabilitation center. Following some hand-reflexology work, a stroke sufferer stood up and turned his arm around, windmill-fashion. "What did you do to John?" asked an employee. In response to our puzzlement, the therapist explained, "He couldn't do that with his paralyzed arm before."

From a gentle press to a focused effort, every move you make as you apply reflexology techniques is a step toward a happier, healthier, and more productive life. Whether your interest is in helping yourself or another, hand reflexology is a life-long skill that can help to maintain self-sufficiency. Relief of common health concerns, improved flexibility of the hands, and overall relaxation… all are possible with hand-reflexology work.

The hands' unique relationship with our bodies links them into our stress mechanism. It is little wonder that wringing one's hands during times of stress is a natural and instinctive attempt to interrupt the tension of the moment. Hands are, after all, integral to our survival responses, ready to spring into action when needed.

Hand-reflexology work provides a simple formula: just as the bank takes our deposits and holds them ready for our use, hand-reflexology techniques contribute to our bank of "wellness standing" ready for the demands of a stressful day. Effective "savers" deposit regularly, building up their balance for a rainy day.

While initial technique application of reflexology addresses current stressors, continued work triggers the healing response for which reflexology is known. One client, for example, found that he could "turn off" his seasonal hay-fever sniffles after two weeks of using a hand-reflexology technique. After this initial period, his sniffle management took less and less time each day.

Hand reflexology offers a bite-sized approach to well-being: the hand is always conveniently available, within our reach when sitting at a red light or during a quiet moment at the end of the day. It is there when we seek to give someone the warmth of touch or a pat of reassurance. Who among us hasn't held a toddler's hand or reached out to comfort an ailing family member? With a little more focus, such touch can turn into the opportunity to trigger the body's own healing powers through hand reflexology's techniques.

The magic of reflexology lies in its empowerment, in the knowledge that by acquiring these skills, one can create change, with one hand helping another. As you read through this book, experience at first hand the power of what you can do for yourself and others.

Barbara K. Kunz

Kevin M. Kunz

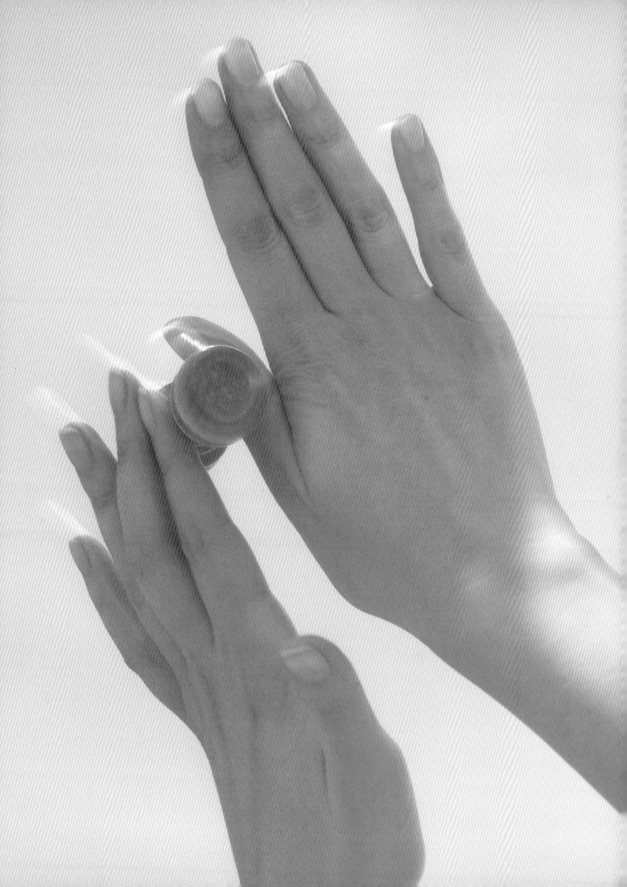

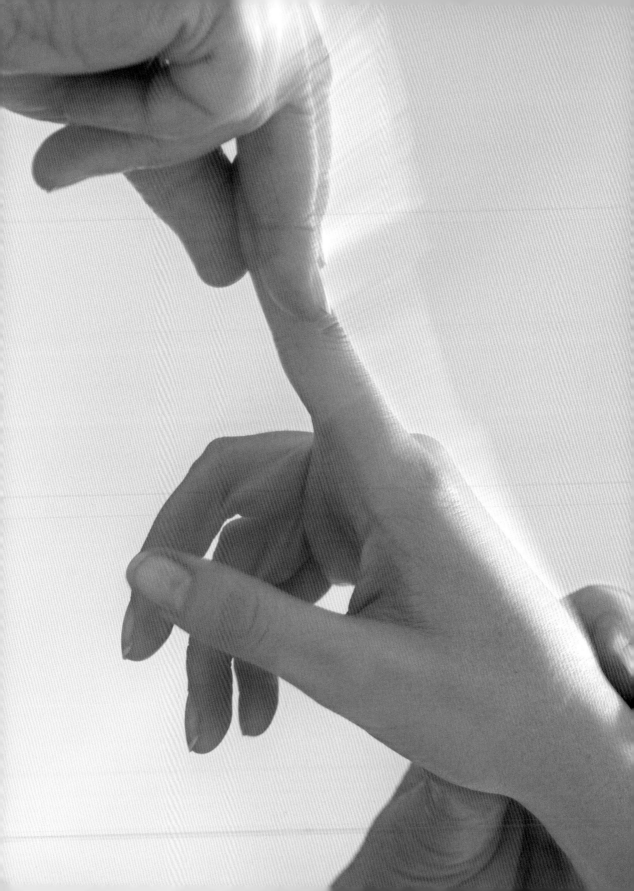

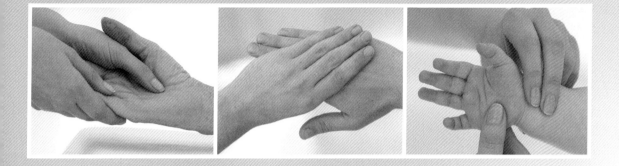

PRINCIPLES OF REFLEXOLOGY

In this ancient therapeutic practice, a variety of pressure techniques are applied to reflex areas of the hands and feet to stimulate responses in corresponding parts of the body. The resulting relaxation has a profoundly beneficial effect on health, preventing disease, reducing pain, and generally improving quality of life. In this chapter, we trace the history of reflexology and examine how and why it works.

THE HISTORY OF REFLEXOLOGY

From ancient times to the present day, reflexology has helped humans maintain health and well-being; its use as a medical practice throughout history is well documented. Although details of the early work are lost in time, archeological clues indicate that reflexology has been rediscovered and reinstated as a health practice time and time again by peoples around the globe seeking to deal with health concerns.

From Egypt to Japan, in China and throughout Asia, artefacts tracing the ancient history of reflexology have been discovered by archaeologists. Although details of the exact principles and techniques are lost to us, the discoveries that have been made testify to the role that this ancient therapy has long played in the health and well-being of people around the world.

REFLEXOLOGY IN ANCIENT EGYPT

Among the oldest relics are pictographs of hand and foot reflexology dating from 2330 BCE, which were discovered at the Tomb of the Physician in Saqqara, Egypt. Carved into stone, these pictographs are included with others showing medical practices of the time.

The Egyptian pictographs are among the oldest known depictions of medical care.

When translated, the hieroglyphs' message resonates with today's reflexologists: "Don't hurt me," to which the physician replies, "I shall act so you praise me." Further references to reflexology span later years in ancient Egyptian history. The victory of Ramses II at Qadesh in 1276 BCE is commemorated with a carving in an obelisk at the temple of Amon at Karnak. A worker is depicted tending to the feet of footsore soldiers

marching to battle. Later, in ancient Egypt, around 50 BCE, Roman emperor Octavian noted Mark Anthony's "pathetic" enslavement to Cleopatra, commenting that he even massaged her feet at dinner parties — giving her an early reflexology treatment.

BUDDHISM AND ASIAN CULTURES

References to the association of feet and hands with health and medicine is found throughout Asia. Some 5,000 years ago in China, the medical text *Hwang Tee Internal Text* included *The Method of Toe Observations*. In Nara, Japan, the *Yakushiji* (Medicine Teacher) Temple includes a bronze statue of the "Healing Buddha" with depictions carved onto the feet and hands. Also on Temple grounds is the *Bussokudo,* a building housing the famous stone bearing the footprint of Buddha (*Bus–soku–seki*). "Medicine Buddha" figures have been found across Asia as well as "Buddha's footprints" dating from 400 BCE. These include similar depictions carved onto the feet and hands. While much of the meaning of these artefacts has been lost in history, their presence testifies to the importance of feet and hands in Buddhism and in cultures across Asia.

UNDERSTANDING THE REFLEX

Why all this interest in reflexology? The answer lies perhaps in reflexology's more recent history. Discoveries made by researchers exploring the nervous system in

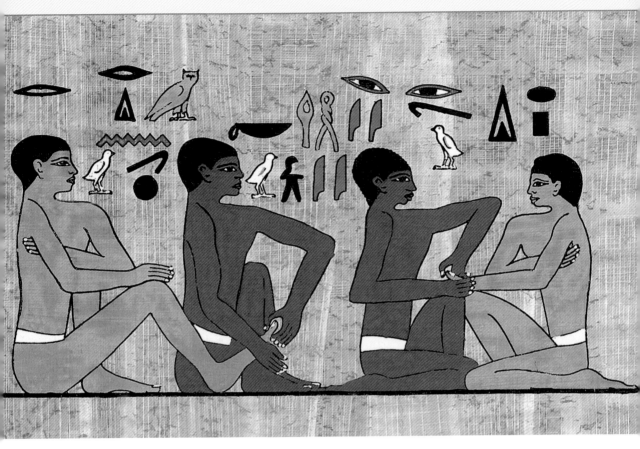

One of the earliest depictions of foot and hand therapy as part of medical care is illustrated in this wall painting from an Egyptian tomb, dating from 2330 BCE.

the mid to late 1800s showed the potential of the reflex as a health tool. As medical doctors in the United Kingdom, Russia, and Germany sought to understand how the nervous system works, alternative schools of thought, research efforts, and published articles were directed toward the reflex, which was seen to offer an opportunity for the provision of health treatment.

Physicians of the late nineteenth century and early twentieth century began to utilize reflex treatment and, in 1917, Russian physician V. M. Bekhterev (1857–1957) coined the term reflexology. British physician Sir Henry Head (1861–1940) developed ideas for the therapeutic uses of reflex actions, mapping the connection between different organs and specific areas of the skin in a model known as "Head's Zones." Reflex zone massage was launched in Germany and, in the United States, Dr. William Fitzgerald (1872–1942) developed his system

The reflex was seen as a window of opportunity for the provision of health treatment.

of "zone therapy," which he used in his eye, ear, nose, and throat practice. His ideas were picked up and developed, most notably by physiotherapist Eunice Ingham (1879–1974), who extended the original simple ten-zone concept, mapping the reflex areas of the hands and feet and their corresponding body parts. Her work of 1938 marks the beginnings of today's reflexology.

The hand is a sensory organ, capable of receiving and communicating sensations such as pressure, stretch, and movement. Hand reflexology uses this ability to send a message of relaxation to the body, resulting in an improved response to daily stresses.

HOW REFLEXOLOGY WORKS

Hands reach out to touch the world, befriending and defending as well as picking up the pieces when necessary, and helping us to survive. Pressure sensors in the hands give us the ability to communicate with others and to manipulate our surroundings, carrying out the daily tasks that make up our lives, and using the tools and equipment that we routinely employ in the performance of those tasks.

At the most fundamental level, the hands are essential to our survival, creating shelter, providing food, and nurturing our young. In times of danger, the hands participate in the overall body reaction that ensures survival. This reaction is commonly known as the "fight or flight response" because it enables the body to gear its internal organs and muscles to respond to either eventuality. The sudden adrenaline surge that enables a person to lift a car following an accident is an example of this extraordinary response to stress.

INTERRUPTING STRESS PATTERNS

The same stress mechanism is also at work as we respond to the demands of the day. When sustained, however, such stress creates wear and tear on the body. According to researcher Hans Selye (1907–1982), 75 percent of all illnesses are stress-related. He argued that interrupting the pattern of stress provides a break in the routine, thereby resolving the wear-and-tear effect of continuous stress. Hand-reflexology work taps into this relationship, interrupting stress and helping to reset the body's overall tension level. As the hand responds to the new sensory experiences of reflexology's pressure

Continuing use of reflexology results in improved response to the stresses of the day.

techniques, the work interrupts patterns of stress and prompts a general, whole-body relaxation response. If practiced sufficiently often, reflexology work not only interrupts stress but also conditions an improved response to it.

Reflexology works as a stress reducer in the nervous system, promoting beneficial effects on the whole body.

Reflexology techniques provide stimulus to pressure sensors of the hands, prompting a reflexive response throughout the body, including on its internal organs. A reflex effect occurs as the body automatically and unconsciously resets its stress mechanism. When reflexology techniques are applied to a specific part of the hand, a specific relaxation response occurs in a corresponding body part: reflexology maps of the hands show this relationship (*see pages 16–19*).

Reflexology work affects the body in three ways: a general relaxation response, a specific reflex effect, and a rejuvenation of the hand itself. It also improves the flexibility of the hand and helps to develop hand awareness, thus lessening the potential for injury. In sum, reflexology works as a stress reducer in the nervous system prompting an effect on the whole body.

REFLEXOLOGY AND ZONES

Reflexology theory is based on zone theory. Just as the meridians of acupuncture link one part of the body to another, so too reflexology links the hand to the body and its organs through a combination of zone charts and hand maps.

Zone theory divides the body into ten zones – one for each finger and toe. Applying pressure to one part of a zone creates an effect along the zone. For example, pressure applied to the index finger creates a reaction, a relaxation response, along zone 2 anywhere in the body. Lateral markers provide a further link between body and hand (*see right*). For example, to influence a body part at the diaphragm in zone 1, pressure is applied to the hand at the diaphragm lateral marker and zone 1 (*see opposite*). This system is further refined as reflexology maps (*see pages 16–19*).

ZONES AND MAPS IN PRACTICE

Reflexologists use the system of zones and hand maps to locate an area on the hand that corresponds to a specific part of the body, in order to address localized stress. For example, our client Twyllah attended the emergency room with her teenage daughter, who was in great pain. Twyllah used her reflexology and zone knowledge to find the part of her daughter's hand that reflected the pain, which she successfully relieved during diagnosis and preparation for an appendectomy.

Reflexologists utilize reflexology maps and zone charts in order to plan their strategy: where to apply technique, how much to apply, and for how long are key questions for a focused approach to prompting the relaxation response. The reflexology map is used as a tool to focus work on specific organs, systems, or functions of the body that may be under stress.

Zone charts

Reflexologists use zone charts similar to the one below to help them locate areas on the hand that correspond to different parts of the body. The body is divided into ten zones and four lateral zones. The lateral markers are: base of the neck, diaphragm (base of the ribcage), the waistline, and base of the pelvis.

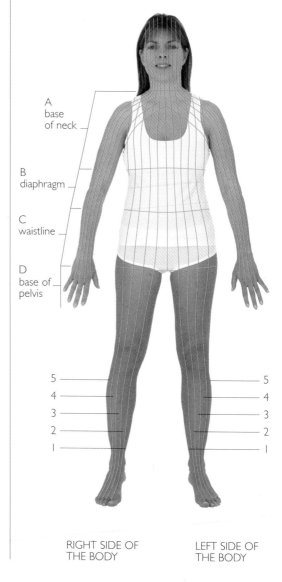

A
base
of neck

B
diaphragm

C
waistline

D
base of
pelvis

5   5
4   4
3   3
2   2
1   1

RIGHT SIDE OF
THE BODY

LEFT SIDE OF
THE BODY

LEFT PALM

RIGHT PALM

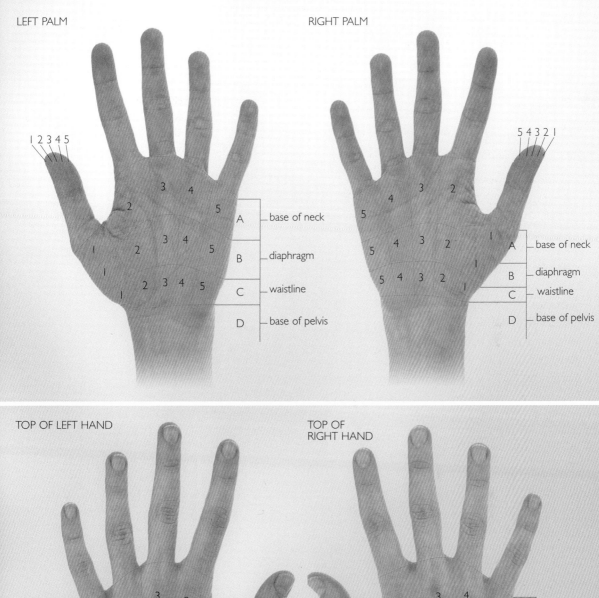

A	base of neck
B	diaphragm
C	waistline
D	base of pelvis

A	base of neck
B	diaphragm
C	waistline
D	base of pelvis

TOP OF LEFT HAND

TOP OF
RIGHT HAND

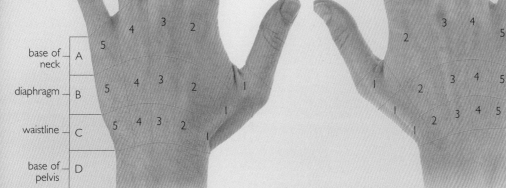

base of neck	A
diaphragm	B
waistline	C
base of pelvis	D

A	base of neck
B	diaphragm
C	waistline
D	base of pelvis

HAND REFLEXOLOGY MAPS

The body's anatomy is mapped onto reflex areas on the fronts and backs of the hands, where the reflex area for the head is located on the tops of the fingers and thumbs. Broken lines indicate where reflex areas overlap.

Left palm

Reflex areas on the left palm correspond to the left side of the body: head and neck areas on the fingers, tailbone near the wrist. The shoulder reflex is on the outside and the spine reflex on the inside.

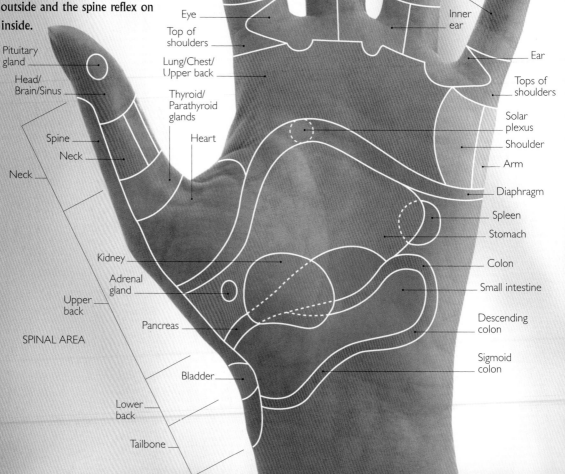

Head/Brain/Sinus

Neck

Eye

Top of shoulders

Inner ear

Ear

Pituitary gland

Head/Brain/Sinus

Lung/Chest/Upper back

Tops of shoulders

Thyroid/Parathyroid glands

Solar plexus

Spine

Heart

Shoulder

Neck

Arm

Neck

Diaphragm

Spleen

Stomach

Kidney

Colon

Adrenal gland

Small intestine

Upper back

Descending colon

Pancreas

SPINAL AREA

Bladder

Sigmoid colon

Lower back

Tailbone

Right palm

Reflex areas on the right palm mirror the right side of the body. Since the two sides of the body have different internal organs, there are differences between the reflexology maps for the right and left hands. For example, the liver reflex area is represented only on the right palm.

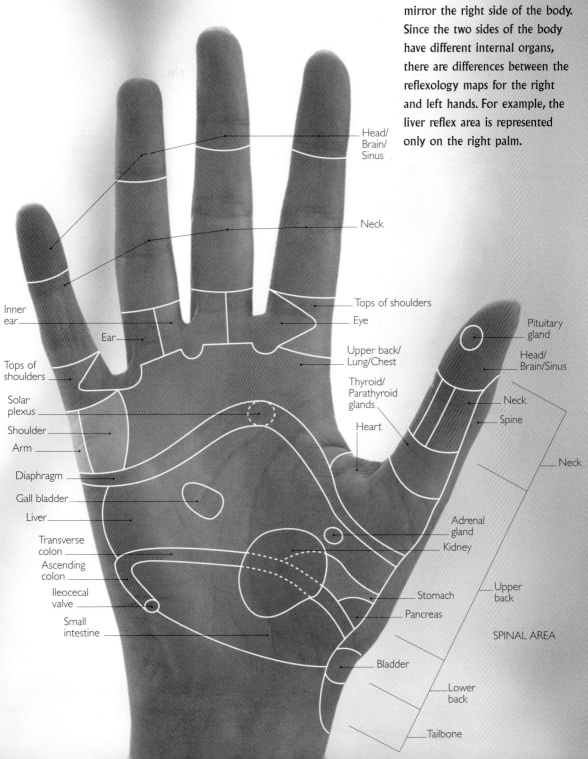

Head/Brain/Sinus

Neck

Tops of shoulders

Eye

Upper back/Lung/Chest

Thyroid/Parathyroid glands

Heart

Pituitary gland

Head/Brain/Sinus

Neck

Spine

Neck

Inner ear

Ear

Tops of shoulders

Solar plexus

Shoulder

Arm

Diaphragm

Gall bladder

Liver

Transverse colon

Ascending colon

Ileocecal valve

Small intestine

Adrenal gland

Kidney

Stomach

Pancreas

Upper back

SPINAL AREA

Bladder

Lower back

Tailbone

Top of left hand

The top of the left hand includes a series of banded reflex areas that relate to the left side of the body, from the left side of the head to the left knee. Reflex areas for the groin, lymph glands, and fallopian tubes can be found on the wrist.

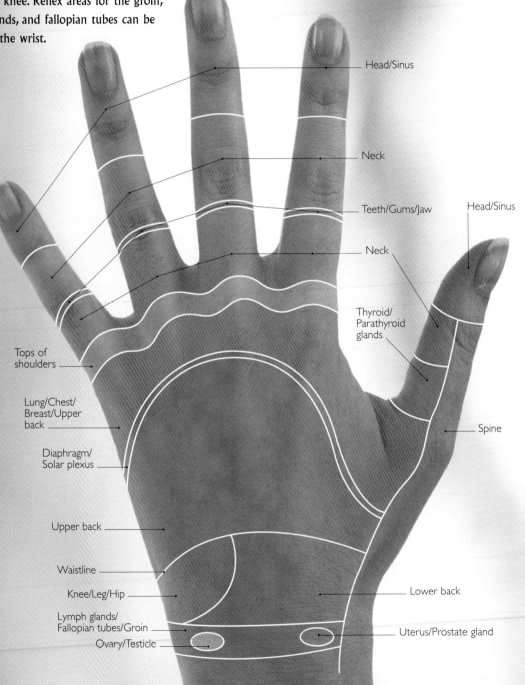

Head/Sinus

Neck

Teeth/Gums/Jaw

Neck

Head/Sinus

Thyroid/
Parathyroid
glands

Tops of
shoulders

Lung/Chest/
Breast/Upper
back

Spine

Diaphragm/
Solar plexus

Upper back

Waistline

Knee/Leg/Hip

Lower back

Lymph glands/
Fallopian tubes/Groin

Ovary/Testicle

Uterus/Prostate gland

Top of right hand

The reflex areas on the right hand correspond to
the body's right side. The "waistline" can be found
at the base of the long bones. Locate the
upper back reflex area just above the
waistline, and below it, the areas
for the lower back, hips, and the
internal organs they protect.

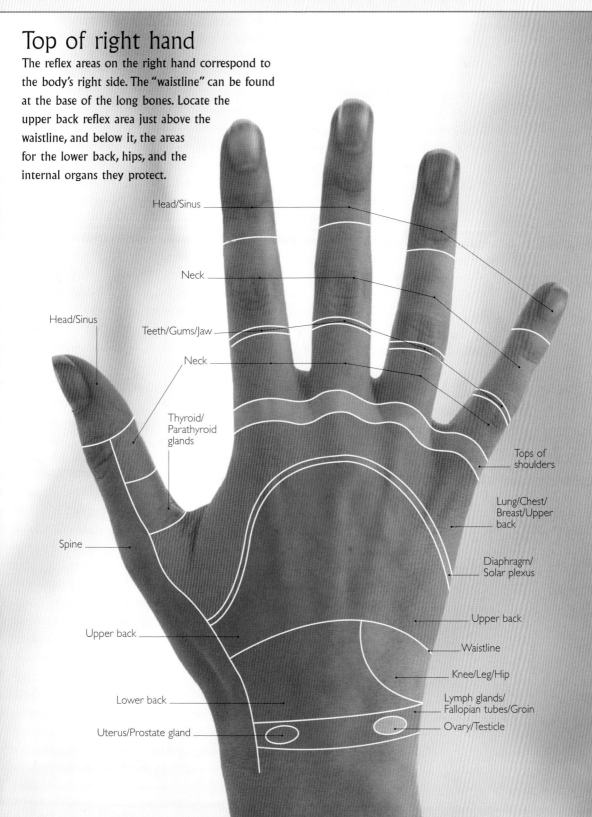

Head/Sinus

Neck

Teeth/Gums/Jaw

Neck

Head/Sinus

Thyroid/
Parathyroid
glands

Spine

Upper back

Lower back

Uterus/Prostate gland

Tops of
shoulders

Lung/Chest/
Breast/Upper
back

Diaphragm/
Solar plexus

Upper back

Waistline

Knee/Leg/Hip

Lymph glands/
Fallopian tubes/Groin

Ovary/Testicle

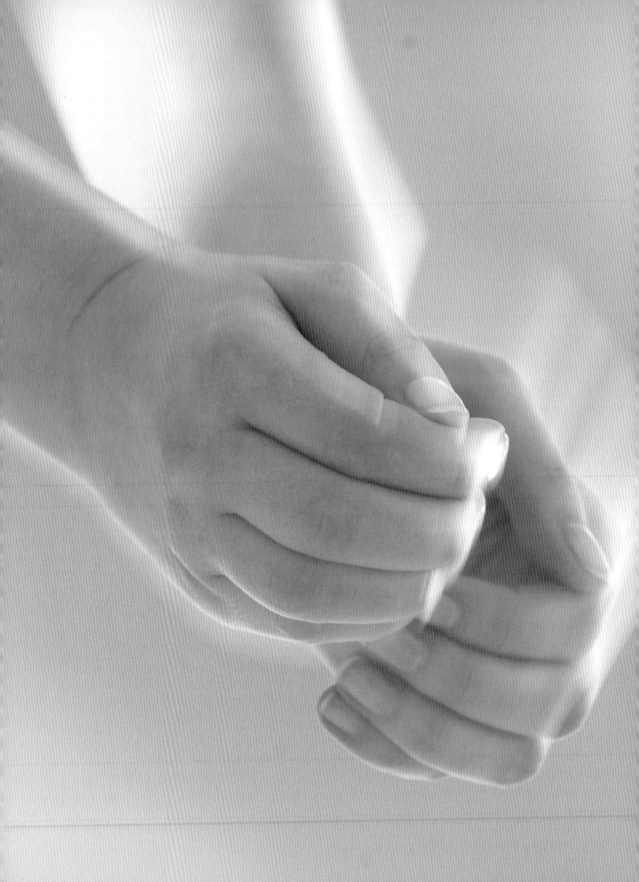

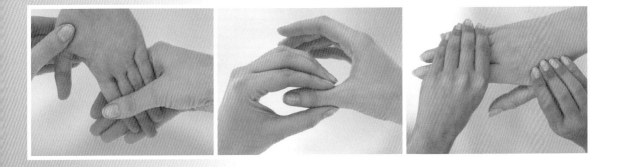

BENEFITS OF REFLEXOLOGY

From infants to senior citizens, reflexology can

benefit people of all ages. By learning how to

use its techniques, you will acquire a skill that can

enable you to improve the health of yourself and

others. This chapter presents research studies that

support the beneficial effects of reflexology, offers

advice on choosing a professional reflexologist, and

provides guidance about what to expect during a

professional reflexology session.

WHY DO PEOPLE USE HAND REFLEXOLOGY?

Hand reflexology is a life skill through which you can create change and improve the quality of life for yourself and others. It offers a safe, effective, and simple method of treating a variety of health problems, as well as a way of easing the stresses of daily life. Learning hand-reflexology skills gives one control over responses to health crises as well as a means of reaching out to others in time of need.

While reflexology success stories are legion (*see pages 32–33*), the opportunity to reach out and help oneself or others with its techniques is unique among health pursuits. Reflexology work provides the practitioner with the ability to help in a meaningful way. Real-life examples of reflexology use include: aiding recovery from the shock of a fall until emergency personnel arrive; helping a concerned relative to comfort a hospice patient; and alleviating chronic sinus problems that are interrupting work. Hand-reflexology skills provide a tool with which to help oneself and others.

POSITIVE STEPS WITH REFLEXOLOGY

Reflexology provides the chance to touch, ease, refresh, calm, relax, and relate. The benefits of hand reflexology are as diverse as the people who use it: from a young soccer player recovering from injury, to a jewelry maker seeking rejuvenation after a day's work, reflexology provides a resource for those who seek well-being. The clear message is that, with reflexology, you can make a difference in your health and in the health of others

Hand reflexology is used because it is effective for a myriad of both general health and specific hand concerns. Research reveals some of the story (*see page 29*), but people in real life use reflexology to address their health concerns. A list of benefits can only begin to describe the stories. One individual wrote us to say: "You saved my life. [Thanks to reflexology] I can now play the piano again." Another letter was from a father whose use of reflexology helped ease the pain and flare-ups of his daughter's chronic disease.

Reflexology is simple, convenient, and portable, allowing you to take positive steps toward health goals throughout the day, no matter where you are or what you are doing. It can be used at odd moments, such as waiting at a red light or watching television, so it can fit in with the busiest schedule. And each application of reflexology technique will contribute to creating a positive impact on your health.

Finally, reflexology is used because it is an activator, a means of actively pursuing health. Reflexology users are launched on a path — in an on-going participation in improving their health and well-being. Knowing that one has the ability to contribute actively provides a sense of control and confidence over responses to life's stresses.

USES & BENEFITS OF HAND REFLEXOLOGY	
Addressing health problems	Creating awareness of the hand and body
Rejuvenating overused or tired hands	Maintaining health
Maintaining manual dexterity	Preventing illness
	Relaxing physically
Aiding recovery from hand injury	Easing pain

Your questions answered

Can reflexology help me with my health problem?

While many have found success with reflexology work, a number of factors are involved, including the nature of the health concern and the general state of health. It is always worth giving reflexology a try as you take positive steps to improve your health; the goal is to lower your stress sufficiently to allow your body to begin to repair itself. The relaxation that is provided by reflexology work is in itself a positive step toward improving health.

How long do I have to work before I can expect results?

How much technique is required to create change varies from person to person. After considering such issues, Chinese researchers suggested that getting results with reflexology depends on how much technique is applied, as well as its frequency, duration, and intensity. How long, how often, and how hard are the variables that can be adjusted for successful reflexology use. For example, light pressure applied frequently was found to work with the elderly, who were sensitive to reflexology work. Based on this idea, individuals with little time to spare might also benefit from short but frequent work. As you work with reflexology, incorporate it into your life so that you do enough to see results.

How can I best use reflexology?

Create reflexology opportunities at home, at work, and when you are out and about – for example, in the car or when using public transport. Use all the reflexology techniques that help to relax your hands, provide overall relaxation, and address your health or hand concerns. Experiment with a variety of mini-sequences to see which techniques work best for you. Make a before and after comparison by

> A client said: "I didn't think anything was happening [as a result of reflexology work], then I suddenly realized that I can now hang clothes on the line without pain."

keeping track of your response to your reflexology work. Before starting, consider how your hand feels, then check whether it feels any different afterward. Does the hand you've worked on feel different from your other hand? Bear in mind how long any different feeling persists. Keep track of how long and how frequently you work before you feel a change.

As your reflexology work continues, you will find that it becomes second nature and you will instinctively reach for the golf ball or apply a reflexology technique in response to the sniffle of an allergy or an aching shoulder.

Can I hurt myself?

Although reflexology work is safe, awareness is important and technique application should be kept within your or your recipient's comfort zone. Overuse can result from the application of technique that is too much, too long, or too hard. If part of the hand feels unduly sensitive to the touch following reflexology work, rest it for a few days before resuming work. Lessen the time and frequency of technique application but, if the hand is still sensitive, stop. Be aware of the potential for overuse when working with tools such as a golf ball, or foot-roller. The hard surface of a tool should be considered for its appropriateness for you before starting to use it.

ADVANTAGES OF HAND REFLEXOLOGY

Hands play a special role in our lives: from giving a simple wave to performing a complex piano piece, our hands are linked to much of what happens every day. And it is these same abilities that make hand reflexology special as well. Taking advantage of the way the hands work, hand reflexology taps easily into your reflexes and uses them to bring about a relaxation response.

The hands are particularly convenient for reflexology work. Whether you are applying reflexology to yourself or another, it is simple to reach out for a hand and apply reflexology technique. One of the clearest advantages of hand reflexology is the ease it offers of playing an active role in reducing stress levels. Because of the easy access, it is possible to apply technique more frequently, thus improving the chance of getting successful results with reflexology work.

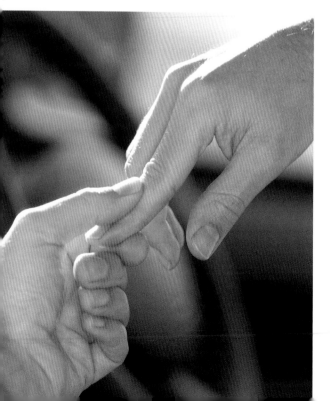

FLEXIBILITY OF HAND REFLEXOLOGY

Working on the hand adds flexibility to reflexology work as there are many occasions when this is more convenient or comfortable for the recipient than foot work. Some people may feel more comfortable having work applied to their hands; others may have suffered a foot injury, which rules out work on the foot.

From the perspective of the person applying the reflexology work, some find hands easier to work on than feet, especially when just starting to learn: we are more familiar with the shape of the hands and with holding and touching the hands of another. There are also physical advantages to working with the hands: many reflex areas, such as those in the webbing of the hands, on the fingers, and on the palms are more accessible on the hand than on the feet.

Hand-reflexology work enhances hand awareness, helping to relax busy hands and prevent hand injury. It also makes us more aware of our hands' capabilities and limits, encouraging us to take care of them. Finally, the clear advantage of hand reflexology is that it improves the workings of the hand, helping aging hands to maintain their function, or those of the musician or keyboard worker to continue earning their living.

Hand-reflexology techniques are simple to apply, providing a convenient and effective means of promoting relaxation and addressing the health concerns of yourself and others.

Your questions answered

Which is better – hand or foot reflexology?

Although both are effective in prompting relaxation and other health benefits, foot reflexology tends to be more widely available and is considered by some people to be more effective. Because feet are usually encased in shoes, they are more protected and thus tend to be more sensitive to the application of reflexology technique. In addition, foot reflexology addresses tired feet, which is a common concern.

Others, however, find that hand reflexology works better for them. It is convenient, addresses the issue of tired or sore hands, and provides a welcome break from the repetitive stress of keyboard-using jobs. In addition, some people simply prefer having their hands worked on – and of course it is more appropriate for self-help.

Which is better: self-help reflexology work or receiving reflexology work?

The clear advantage of self-help reflexology is the convenience of working on oneself at any time, making frequency of technique application possible. Receiving reflexology from another, however, has the advantage of touch, which can promote a deeper relaxation effect.

Questions to ask yourself

There is usually a specific reason why people turn to reflexology, so make sure you know what that is in order to focus your efforts. To help, consider the following statements and see what rings true:

Are your hands tired?

Do you find yourself saying:
My hands hurt/I work with my hands all day/I am aware of the tension in my hands all the time.

Do you have a hand concern?

Do you find yourself saying:
I have had a hand operation, injury, and/or hand problem and I want to take better care of my hands.

Do you have a health concern?

Do you find yourself saying:
My shoulder is aching/My digestion bothers me/My back hurts all the time.

Are you concerned about stress?

Do you find yourself saying:
I've been stressed at home/work/I'm on a deadline and I'm looking to reduce my stress level.

Are you seeking ways to maintain your health and prevent problems?

Do you find yourself saying:
I'm interested in taking care of myself/I'd rather spend the money to reduce tension now than suffer from stress-related conditions later.

Do you like to seek out positive contributions to your well-being?

Do you find yourself saying:
I like to do good things for my health and I look for things I can add to my program.

Do you like to pamper yourself?

Do you find yourself saying:
I treat myself to these little luxuries.

Are you a fan of hand reflexology?

Do you find yourself saying:
I like having my hands worked on because I like the way they feel afterward.

Do you need a little pep-me-upper?

Do you find yourself saying:
I know I'm pushing my body but I have things to do.

REFLEXOLOGY FOR EVERYONE

Reflexology can offer a helping hand to everyone, regardless of their age, occupation, or current state of health. From the soothing touch offered to an infant, relief of stress for the keyboard worker, or a feeling of control over falls offered to the elderly, reflexology helps to meet specific health goals, maintain health and well-being, and enhance the quality of life for each and every one of us.

For both the healthy and the not-so-healthy, the reflexology experience provides a psychological comfort zone where inner thoughts can be shared and a sense of relaxation evolves with the application of the techniques.

WORKING WITH BABIES

Babies are a natural for reflexology, benefiting from a light touch. Working these tiny hands can encourage the development of nervous system pathways from the hand to the brain. While the waving of hands and feet in the newborn exhibits the beginnings of a positioning awareness, movement intelligence can be enhanced with a few gentle stimulations of the hand.

We've talked with many parents who report their delight when reflexology deals successfully with their little ones' common problems. One friend was amazed to find that a few gentle touches could lull her baby to sleep. Another found that reflexology alleviated the distress of her infant as their plane was landing. Others have used a gentle press to help a colicky baby (*see page 110*). Comforting a sick infant with a few simple presses allows you to communicate your care with a soothing touch.

The gentle touch of reflexology soothes fretful infants, helping them to relax.

HELPING CHILDREN

More than one parent has told us how reflexology has helped them connect with their children. A common story is that when faced with a child who can't sleep, doesn't feel good, or has a tummyache, the parents have tried a little reflexology work. Soon they find the child plopping down next to them on the couch and sticking a foot or hand in their laps any time they need comfort. As the child grows, such a scenario becomes a regular moment of quiet communication. The application of reflexology technique helps parent and child cope with life's ups and downs in a natural way, smoothing the physical transitions at different stages of development as well as stimulating the brain.

Staff at a school in London confirm this, reporting that providing reflexology services for students and their families "helps bring children closer to parents with whom they previously had little relationship."

Reflexology techniques help parent and child cope with life's ups and downs.

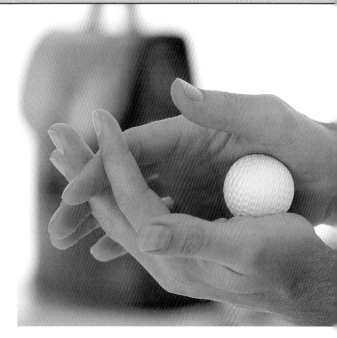

Office workers whose keyboard use results in tired, sore hands can benefit from learning a few self-help techniques. Keep a golf ball in your drawer for a simple workout.

OLDER PEOPLE

Not only does reflexology work help ease the health concerns of the elderly, but the experience of a little touch and a listening ear can provide a highlight in their day. Research shows the positive impact on common health concerns, including decrease in pain, improved heart, kidney, and bowel function, and reduction in stress. Reflexology work also improves quality of life in issues such as having the flexibility to fasten buttons and open doors, and maintaining an independent life for as long as possible. A study of cobblestone-mat walking – an exercise popular in China, in which participants walk barefoot on a mat with a smooth, undulating, cobblestone-like surface – showed that its use improves balance when walking, improving stability and decreasing the likelihood of falls. Some of our favorite reflexology stories are of seniors whose reflexology work has improved both their health and that of others. For example, a retired teacher used reflexology to improve the flexibility in his fingers, then went on to help his wife who had experienced a stroke.

IN THE WORKPLACE

Reflexology plays an important role in keeping hands happy in the workplace. Feel-good dessert techniques (*see pages 60–65*) provide a respite for hands that are tired from keyboarding. Reflexology work also provides relaxation to the neck, shoulders, and arms through the application of technique to corresponding reflex areas on the hands. Such work lowers stress in the body and lessens the potential for wear and tear and even of injury. This work is important, since studies have shown a relationship between overall stress and keyboard-related hand concerns such as carpal tunnel syndrome.

TREATING ELDERLY PEOPLE

Touch is perhaps the aspect of reflexology that is most enjoyed by older people. A relaxing hand reflexology session, accompanied by a few moments of conversation, can greatly improve quality of life. As well as general relaxation techniques, you may wish to add specific techniques to address particular health concerns (see pages 120–153). For example, to address sluggish digestive processes, apply the thumb-walking technique to the colon reflex area (see pages 72–73).

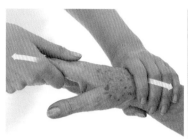

The finger-pull (see page 63) promotes relaxation and improves flexibility, so start the session by gently applying this dessert to each finger and thumb in turn. Be careful to stay within the client's comfort zone.

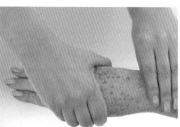

End the session with the squeeze (see page 65), which uses gentle pressure to relax the whole hand. Gently and firmly squeeze the hand several times, repositioning and then repeating along the length of the hand.

PREGNANT WOMEN

Research shows what many have already discovered for themselves: reflexology work helps women to have easier pregnancies, quicker and less painful deliveries, and more success with breastfeeding their infants. As the body changes throughout pregnancy, reflexology work helps with common concerns such as backache, aching neck, swollen feet, and nausea.

The stress of pregnancy and delivery may not end with the birth. Post-partum depression is a reality for some women. A friend who recognized the signs of unhappiness in her niece after she gave birth utilized her reflexology skills as well as an understanding ear to help the new mother through a difficult time.

PEOPLE WITH PHYSICAL DISABILITIES

Touch is frequently an element missing in the lives of people with physical disabilities, so reflexology's hands-on communication can bring a particularly valuable type of comfort. In addition, reflexology helps interrupt stress, lessening energy demands for handicapped individuals who expend 30 percent more energy in the tasks they perform throughout the day. Most of all,

reflexology provides the possibility for improved quality of life for those with physical disabilities. Our friend Alice, for example, worried that doctors' predictions would be borne out – that her daughter would never live independently following a car crash that resulted in paralysis and head injury. The concerned mother learned reflexology and began work on her daughter, who eventually returned to her career as a teacher, and to independent living.

THOSE WITH SERIOUS ILLNESS

Reflexology work gives one the ability to connect with those suffering from a serious illness, injury, or surgery. With reflexology skills, visitors can also be care-givers when their loved ones are in hospital. Instead of sitting around feeling useless, you can be helping. With the gift of touch in your reflexology work, you can demonstrate to the recipient how much you care. Applying a few hand desserts or techniques to a patient in hospital does more than flowers or candy ever can. As one study found, patients who received reflexology from their relatives felt less abandoned and the family members felt satisfied that they could aid the loved one.

REFLEXOLOGY RESEARCH

Research supports the beneficial uses of reflexology work: studies show that reflexology techniques affect the body, helping it to function better, easing pain, and hastening recovery from illness. In addition, researchers have established plausible reasons to explain these effects. In studies around the world, researchers have demonstrated the potential of reflexology for improving quality of life.

Researchers in Israel found that reflexology achieves positive results in multiple sclerosis patients, alleviating motor, sensory, and urinary symptoms (2003). American researchers discovered reflexology to be an "effective, inexpensive, low-risk, flexible, and easily applied strategy for post-operative pain management" (2005).

Also in the US, researchers working with hospitalized breast cancer patients found reflexology to be successful in the management of pain, nausea, and anxiety (2000).

Another study of patients with breast cancer reported positive results in alleviating pain and anxiety, finding too that reflexology offers a "simple technique for human touch which can be performed anywhere, requires no special equipment, is non-invasive, and does not interfere with patients' privacy."

Quality of life improved for senior citizens using a reflexology cobblestone mat. Researchers found that reflexology helped seniors in "promoting and maintaining functional mobility and overall health status" (US, 2003, 2005).

In addition, research provides evidence that reflexology work can create a physical response of choice. In a study by researchers in Austria, reflexology work on the kidney reflex area was found to affect blood flow to the kidneys (1999). A further study by those researchers (2001) showed increased blood flow to the intestines following reflexology work applied to

Research demonstrates that reflexology work can create a physical response on specific organs of the body.

the corresponding reflex area. A researcher in India who found that reflexology reduced post-surgical pain theorized that the pressure signal of reflexology technique application successfully blocked out pain signals, thus alleviating pain (2006).

EXPLAINING REFLEXOLOGY

These studies may explain why reflexology works. The improvement in blood flow to the kidneys noted above could explain why other studies found that treatment for kidney stones proceeds more quickly with reflexology work (1996). Similarly, improved blood flow to the intestines could explain why reflexology work was found to ease constipation (China, 1994).

In Singapore, researchers tracking reflexology work with an EEG test found that it triggers the same brain-wave pattern as is found in those resting in a deeply relaxed state (2005). Further studies show that reflexology prompts normalization of the body's organs. A British study (1997) and a study in Singapore (2005) both demonstrate improvement on heart function.

REFLEXOLOGY IN MEDICAL CARE

Research studies demonstrating the efficacy of reflexology work have led to its adoption in medical care, where it is proving to be a valuable adjunct to standard practice. Patients in hospices, those receiving treatment for cancer and other life-threatening illnesses, the elderly, and pregnant women have all found their quality of life enhanced by the application of reflexology work.

With growing research evidence of the benefits of reflexology work in medical care, and with so many patients themselves requesting this service, medical establishments are increasingly making reflexology treatment available to patients.

PROVISION OF SERVICES

Studies demonstrating that reflexology eases nausea, vomiting, and fatigue in breast cancer patients undergoing chemotherapy has prompted the addition of reflexology services at many facilities, including the M. D. Anderson Cancer Center in Houston, Texas. Hospices across the United Kingdom now utilize reflexology as a way of helping to provide patients and their families with more dignity, choice, and control.

Hospices are using reflexology to provide dignity, choice, and control for patients and families.

Reflexology work in such settings helps to improve a patient's quality of life, offering practical ways of coping with life-threatening illness, providing comfort, and enhancing both the patient's and the carer's sense of emotional, physical, and spiritual well-being. An audit of all hospices in Scotland found that half of these establishments provide reflexology services, with

respondents in the study reporting an improved quality of life, through a reduction in both physical and emotional symptoms. Also in Scotland, community nurses are now using reflexology to manage fecal incontinence and constipation in children.

In Eire, at the National Maternity Hospital in Dublin, reflexology is being used to ease the experiences of pregnancy and birthing, as well as for treating pre- and post-natal depression and gynecological conditions such as endometriosis and premenstrual tension (PMS).

In the United States, many medical, nursing, and pharmacy schools are incorporating the study of complementary medicine, reflexology, and other therapies into their curriculum. For example, the University of Pennsylvania's Presbyterian Medical Center in Philadelphia plans to train medical staff to develop personalized therapy plans that include reflexology, with

---

USES OF REFLEXOLOGY IN MEDICAL CARE

Researchers have demonstrated that reflexology can play a valuable role in medical care, easing symptoms, relieving pain, and enhancing quality of life:

Pain relief and improved quality of life for the elderly.

Relief of symptoms for patients undergoing chemotherapy.

Palliative care for hospice patients.

Quality of life for those diagnosed with multiple sclerosis.

the goal of decreasing patient stress, pain, and anxiety. Reflexology services are already being provided at clinics associated with medical schools, such as the Outpatient Services at the University of Pittsburgh Medical Center for Integrative Medicine.

SELF-CARE STRATEGY

The application of reflexology as a self-care strategy has been suggested by researchers both for individuals seeking to alleviate their own symptoms and for family members wishing to help and comfort their loved ones. Researchers working with the elderly found reflexology to be efficacious and suggest that it be used "to develop simple, convenient, and readily accessible exercise programs that will reduce health problems and improve the quality of life of the aging population" (US, 2003).

Use of reflexology as a form of self-care provides a means for family, friends, and individuals themselves to improve quality of life while undergoing medical treatment. Everyone is familiar with the comfort bestowed by the touch of a reassuring hand. Reflexology provides such an opportunity, but much more as well. For

Reflexology can reduce health problems and improve quality of life of the aging population.

example, reaching out to pat a hand after surgery is a natural response, but giving a hand rub may do more, easing pain as well as giving comfort (Korea, 2004). Similarly, a study of people diagnosed with multiple sclerosis — a disease for which medicine has few answers — found that using reflexology improved quality of life (Israel, 2003).

HELPING THE ELDERLY

In the United States, researchers from the Oregon Research Institute (2003, 2005) studied the effects of reflexology cobblestone-mat walking by elderly participants and found that they experienced considerable improvements in many areas of their life, including performance of daily activities, less pain, and lowered blood pressure. Such studies confirm the value of reflexology work in reducing health problems and improving quality of life of the aging population.

The reassuring touch of another's hands is not just comforting to those undergoing medical care; when combined with reflexology skills, it is also therapeutic.

SUCCESS STORIES

Any reflexology enthusiast can tell you his or her favorite success story – but the bottom line is always the same: aid, comfort, and support was provided by reflexology work. These stories illustrate why reflexology has become such an important part of many people's lives.

When you read these short case studies, you will get some idea of how reflexology can enrich your life and that of others. Why not put yourself in a position to experience the successful use of reflexology? Use the techniques on yourself in order to become familiar with the reflex areas, their use, and the proper application of techniques. Try it on others who are interested. Find a reflexology buddy so you, too, can be on the receiving end of reflexology work. Or consider treating yourself to professional reflexology services.

DEVELOPING YOUR SKILLS

Each piece of reflexology work is a step in a positive direction. As you can see from the case studies, reflexology work produces immediate results in some situations; in others, degrees of success come over time. As your reflexology work progresses, consider each interruption of stress to be a positive result in itself, as is the rewarding sense of empowerment and self-control.

As you get results and discover your own success stories, you will become more and more tempted to make reflexology a part of your life: a golf ball in your desk drawer for self-help, work on family and friends, advice about what to do for a health concern when asked, and using reflexology for your health concerns.

Case studies
Combating workplace pollution

Sally had breathing difficulties following years of exposure to chemicals and aerosols in the course of her work as a cosmetologist. Looking for respite, she sought reflexology services. Her breathing eased and, over time, the problem was eliminated.

Getting results

Our niece was being wheeled into the delivery room when she suddenly realized that she did not have her golf ball to hand. Since she had found that using a golf-ball technique had helped relieve some problems during pregnancy, she asked a nurse to bring the ball to her. The staff were surprised at the ease of her delivery. Later, on a plane trip, when her infant son was fussing as the plane came in to land, she used a reflexology technique to help him relax and overcome his discomfort at the change in altitude and pressure.

Averting shock following trauma

Our friend Alex's eagerly anticipated hiking experience in the forest had gone awry when he fell down a cliff, sustaining serious injuries to his legs and pelvis. As his fellow-hikers transported him to medical help several hours away, they used reflexology techniques to help ward off the threat of shock. The emergency-room doctor was surprised by Alex's condition, commenting that he wouldn't have expected to see someone who had undergone such trauma to be in such good shape.

The knowledge that one can have a positive effect on one's own health can only provide an emotional uplift.

Improve quality of life

A client, suffering from partial paralysis as a result of a debilitating illness, had one request – that he regain use of his hand sufficiently to use the remote control for the television. He explained that, because of his condition, watching television was his main source of entertainment. Reflexology work helped make it possible for him to use the remote again.

Touch

Another client, a retired professional, would come to her reflexology appointments wearing her mink jacket, even bringing a special hanger for it. She did not have any physical complaints but seemed to relish the attention and contact.

Sally found that her breathing difficulties, caused by work-place pollution, eased and the problem was eliminated.

Recovery

Recovery from a life-threatening condition had left client Bob depleted, discouraged, and dependent on expensive medication. As his reflexology work progressed, his color improved, he reported feeling better, his medication was withdrawn by the doctor, and he now reports feeling good.

Eating anxieties

Client Ann sought help from reflexology for her eating disorder. Even advice from experts had failed to help her anxiety about food. What did help was the relaxing effect of reflexology work. As the work progressed, her anxiety at the dinner table diminished, her body awareness improved, as did her eating habits.

Doctors were surprised to see our friend Alex in such good shape following a cliff fall and lengthy delay in getting medical help. Colleagues had used reflexology techniques to ward of the possibility of shock.

Relieving asthma

Katharine's asthma attacks were no longer being relieved by the medication that she had taken for years, and her attacks were increasingly wakening her in the night as she struggled to breathe. We showed Katharine how to apply a self-help technique to the adrenal gland reflex area. She was delighted to discover that by putting this technique into practice, she was able to control her asthma attacks and breathe freely.

Easing tired feet

Maria's work as a waitress in a busy restaurant meant that she was on her feet for hours on end each day. The stress on her body was manifesting itself not just in tired feet, but also in headaches, backache, and general fatigue. Reflexology sessions have not only eased Maria's immediate symptoms, but shown her that by obtaining total relaxation, her general health and well-being are significantly improved. She has also learned self-help techniques that she can put into practice throughout the day, whenever she finds a spare moment.

Applying a self-help reflexology technique helped Katharine deal with asthma attacks when medication no longer worked.

VISITING A REFLEXOLOGIST

When you visit a professional reflexologist, you should expect to receive the same professional attitude as with any other healthcare professional. After a few preliminary questions, you may be seated on a reclining chair or massage table. For work on the feet, you will have to remove your shoes and socks, but will be offered a towel or blanket to cover bare legs.

A reflexology session can last from 30 minutes to an hour in length. A professional reflexologist will apply technique to the whole hand in a systematic manner, with additional emphasis on reflex areas that correspond to your specific health and hand concerns. Desserts or "feel-good" techniques will also be applied. The pressure should be within your comfort level: if it hurts at all, it should "hurt good" and not seem threatening in any way. If you feel any discomfort, ask the reflexologist to lighten pressure or to stop work on that area.

DURING THE SESSION

Expect a professional reflexologist to apply sufficient and appropriate technique to give you a sense of relaxation. He or she will also give you feedback during the session as they assess different reflex areas. The reflexologist, in turn, should listen to your concerns, paying attention to your likes and dislikes and to your comments on your experience of the session.

EVALUATING YOUR EXPERIENCE

Assess results during and after the session. When work is complete on one hand, ask for a moment to reflect. Flex your hands, noticing whether or not there is a feeling of relaxation in that hand as well as a difference in feeling between the two hands.

After completion of the session, consider whether or not you feel an overall sense of relaxation. Consider, too, if the session included unexpected additions, such as explanations about reflexology, the location of reflex areas, and advice on self-help techniques.

If you feel any discomfort during your reflexology session, ask the therapist to lighten the pressure.

Your questions answered

When choosing a reflexologist

In seeking a skilled reflexologist, consider the reflexologist's ability to get results for you. Reflexology work involves unique abilities: proficiency is created by the sum total of the reflexologist's experience and skills, so look for a reflexologist who has had sufficient hands-on experience to master technique skills. Check also that he or she has worked successfully with health and hand concerns.

Every profession has its enthusiasts, individuals who are immersed in the work they do. If you find such a reflexologist, you may have found someone whose passion for the field is fueled by results.

When you start looking for a reflexologist, ask around for the name of a practitioner with a reputation for getting results. Try a sample session to see if their's is a technique application you like, to see if it fits with what you're looking for. Ask them questions to ascertain their proficiency.

When opting for a reflexology session, stay aware of your own tastes and keep in mind the reasons why you decided to seek reflexology work. Whether it is tired hands, a health concern, or some other reason, make your interests known to the reflexologist to ensure that you receive the appropriate treatment.

Evaluate your reflexology session both during and afterward: does the hand that has been worked on feel any different? Did you feel an overall sense of relaxation at the end of the session?

Questions to ask the reflexologist

When you call to make the appointment, ask for clarification about fees, forms of payment, and the length of sessions. Ask about the reflexologist's experience and training. You will want to know how many years he or she has been practicing. Also, you will also want to know that the reflexologist has completed a proper course of study in reflexology.

Do you provide other services or sell products?

If the answer is yes, you will have to consider how much of this individual's professional practice is devoted to the application of reflexology. If he or she is only a part-time reflexologist, it does raise a concern as to whether his or her experience and focus are sufficient to achieve results for you.

What kind of services do you provide?

Ask the reflexologist about the nature of his or her services, and whether he or she works on hands or feet. Some reflexologists are not educated or experienced in hand reflexology. Ask also whether he or she offers sessions using cream, oil, or lotion: the question is whether the practitioner is providing reflexology or massage services. You should look for the service that matches what you are comfortable with and what is effective for you.

How many sessions do I need in order to see results?

You should feel that your hand is relaxed as soon as work on it is completed, and by the end of a session, you should feel generally relaxed. After two or three sessions, you should start seeing results, such as easing of a particular health concern – but remember that the longer you have had a problem, the longer it will take to see results.

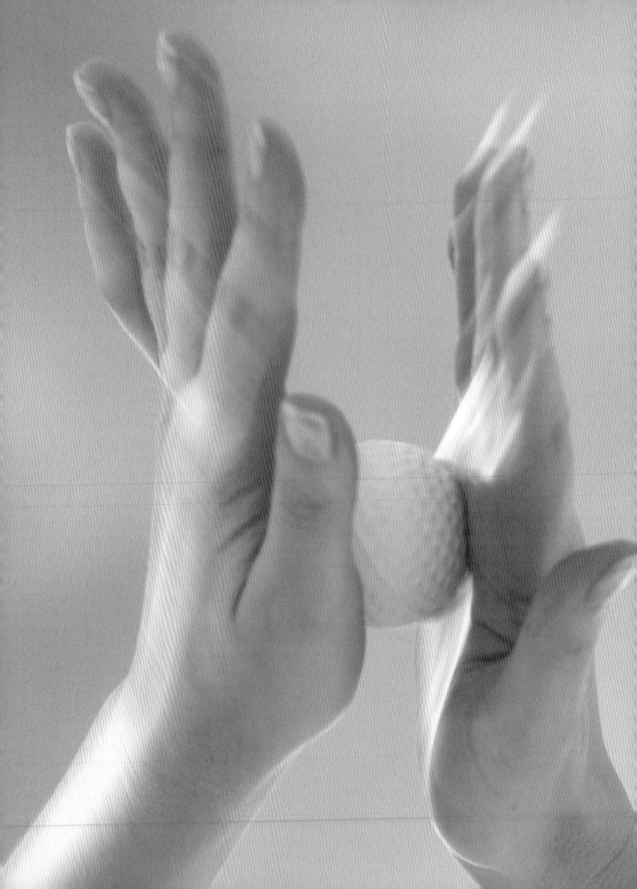

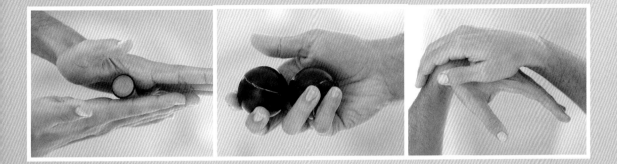

TAKING CARE OF HANDS

Constantly in use throughout the day, our hands

encounter many stresses and strains that can lead

to problems. In this chapter, you'll find techniques

for relaxing those hard-working hands, as well

as tips on breaking up the stress of repetitive

daily tasks such as typing. We also explain how

ergonomics can help keep your hands happy

by looking at the design of tools and equipment

and the way you use them in your daily life.

ANATOMY OF THE HAND

The versatility and dexterity of the hands result from their unique anatomy and physiology. Each hand is made up of 27 bones (making up one quarter of the body's total), connected by muscles and ligaments and served by blood, nerve, and sensory receptors. All of these make possible movements intrinsic to our daily lives, such as oppositional thumb, rotating wrist, and gripping strength.

The hand is undoubtedly the most versatile part of the skeleton, enabling us to grasp and manipulate objects; capable of carrying heavy weights, and supplied with extensive sensory capabilities. To consider the complexity of the hand's movements, think about bending your little finger. This simple act requires an orchestrated effort from brain to finger and back again, all the time activating a complicated arrangement of muscles, tendons, and nerves.

THE BONES OF THE HAND

Of the 200–210 bones in the human body, 54 are in the hands, 27 in each. These include the phalanges (the bones of the fingers), the metacarpals (the long bones), and the carpals (the small bones of the wrist). Bone is living tissue, growing and changing throughout life, and constantly being renewed. During childhood, cartilage turns into bone in a regular sequence. Bones are given rigidity and hardness by minerals such as calcium and phosphorus, but give up these minerals in times of shortage in other parts of the body – hence the importance of having a regular supply in our diets. Bone marrow, which fills the cavities

A complex arrangement of bones, muscles, tendons, and nerves enables the hands to perform their intricate tasks.

Hands are rich in sensitive nerve endings, making them particularly receptive to reflexology work.

in the bones, is a soft, fatty substance that produces most of the body's blood cells.

Of particular importance in hand movement is a group of muscles responsible for the thumb, whose movements are involved in 50 percent of all the hand's activities. The thumb's ability to work in opposition to the fingers is noteworthy as it is this ability that makes possible actions such as grasping and manipulation. Holding a piece of paper, gripping a pen, or working with a screwdriver would be difficult if not impossible without this ability. To check this out for yourself, try to pick up a mug or a ball without involving your thumb.

THE HAND'S MOVEMENTS

Complex and intricate hand movements are achieved by activating the small muscles that are contained entirely within the hand, as well as the much larger muscles and tendons in the forearm. Consider, for example, the action of the thumb when thumb-walking (*see page 54*): as you apply the technique, which involves making only very small movements of the first joint of the thumb, you can observe the activity of the muscles in the forearm as the thumb moves.

The bones of the hand

These consist of the bones of the wrist (the carpals), the long, straight bones of the palm (the metacarpals), and the bones of the fingers (the phalanges). The 14 phalanges are arranged in jointed, continuous segments that enable independent or united action. Bony support is provided to the palm of the hand by the five metacarpals. The eight carpal bones form the heel of the hand, joining the bones of the forearm to create the wrist.

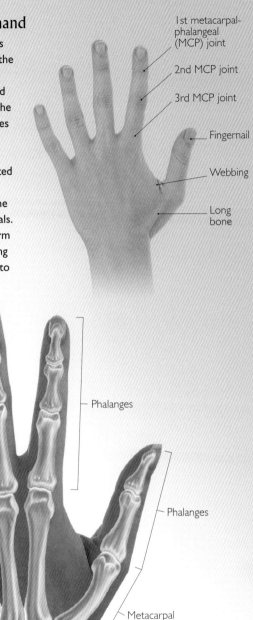

1st metacarpal-phalangeal (MCP) joint

2nd MCP joint

3rd MCP joint

Fingernail

Webbing

Long bone

Phalanges

Phalanges

Metacarpal ("long") bones

Metacarpal ("long") bones

Carpals

LEFT HAND

LOOKING AT THE HAND

An examination of the hand's appearance can reveal quite a lot about the health, age, and lifestyle of an individual. The fingernails, in particular, can be viewed as a window into health, their thin, transparent structure providing a glance into the blood vessels that flow under them.

The quality of the nails is an indicator of health and age. While vertical ridges come with aging, horizontal white lines may result from taking certain drugs while the nails were forming; or they may follow an infectious disease or recent surgery. Some changes, such as little white spots, can result from low-grade infections.

All-white nails may indicate liver problems, while nails that are half pink and half white may point to kidney disorders. Signs of diabetes include a yellowish tint and a slight pink coloring at the base of the nail. Yellow coloring can indicate lung illness, such as tuberculosis and asthma, and fungal infections. A whitish color may be indicative of chronic hepatitis or cirrhosis, while pale color may indicate anemia. Bluish nails may be a sign of circulation problems – this color has been connected to chronic lung disorders such as emphysema or asthma. It may also indicate heart failure or exposure to toxins such as copper or silver.

Nail color isn't the only indicator of health: brittle nails may indicate dehydration, especially if they split. Breaking, splitting fingernails could be a sign of thyroid problems, while misshapen nails may be a sign of arthritis or nutritional deficiency.

ERGONOMICS AND THE HANDS

Your hands perform so many essential tasks that you probably can't imagine life without them. It is therefore important that you take good care of them, not only through the regular use of hand reflexology, but also by taking action to prevent hand strain and injury in the first place. By considering the ergonomics, or optimum positioning, of your hands you can ensure their well-being.

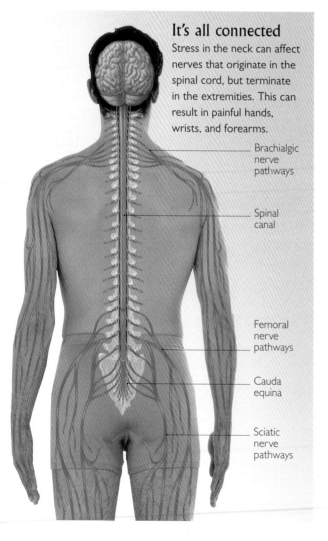

It's all connected

Stress in the neck can affect nerves that originate in the spinal cord, but terminate in the extremities. This can result in painful hands, wrists, and forearms.

Brachialgic nerve pathways

Spinal canal

Femoral nerve pathways

Cauda equina

Sciatic nerve pathways

WHAT IS ERGONOMICS?

Ergonomics is the study of the relationship between workers and their environment, especially the equipment they use. Ergonomists examine the interplay between the design and body positioning in order to prevent the problems and disabilities that may arise as a result of physical stress and the strain of repetitive work.

A relatively new discipline, ergonomics (which is sometimes known as biotechnology) emerged during the Second World War as a proliferation of technological innovations produced new systems and machinery that would have to be operated by workers. These systems were among the first to be designed to take into account how people would use them, and the advent of this study made it possible for them to be manned safely and effectively.

WHY IS IT IMPORTANT?

Ergonomics applies to the whole body, but the hard-working hand, in particular, faces innumerable stresses and strains. The repetitive nature of everyday life means that the same hand muscles, tendons, and ligaments often get used over and over again in repetitive

It is not just typists who are at risk: any repetitive movement can damage the hands.

patterns. It almost goes without saying that those parts of the hand can become strained and overworked. It is not just typists and manual workers who are at risk: any manual activity that involves repetitive movement, including knitting, sewing, playing a musical instrument, or participation in sports – can damage the hands. If left untreated, this pattern of overuse will take its toll. For professionals who habitually use keyboards, for example, repetitive strain injuries such as tendonitis or carpal tunnel syndrome (*see pages 148–149*) can cause severe pain and may even end a career.

WHAT SHOULD I DO?

The symptoms of conditions such as carpal tunnel syndrome, including pain, numbness, and tingling in the hands, result from compression at the wrist of the median nerve. Research indicates that general overall stress and body positioning are also causative factors. If you are experiencing pain, particularly in your hands or forearms, you should consider changing the way you

Consider changing the way you position your body (including your hands) when you work.

position your body (including your hands) when you work. For example, if you work at a desk, how high (or low) is your seat? If you use a computer, must you always reach across your desk to grasp the mouse? And how do you position your wrists over the keyboard as you type? Any of these factors may be contributing to the pain you are experiencing, if your work station is not properly arranged, and a simple change of body position could prevent further strain.

Check your hand position when using equipment such as kitchen knives (see top, right), keyboards (see center, right), and tennis raquets (see bottom, right).

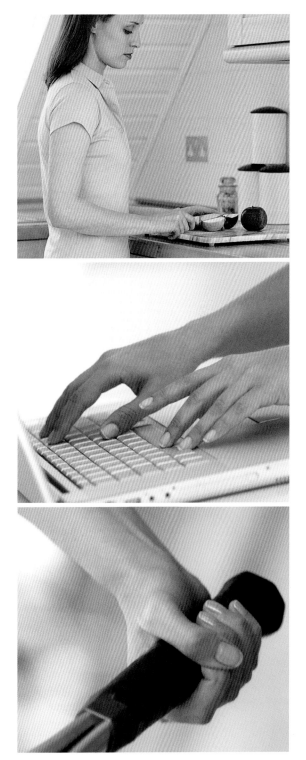

As using a keyboard becomes ever-more common in the workplace and at home, stress-related hand injuries are also increasing. Applying reflexology techniques to relax the hands can play a vital role in preventing problems.

HANDS: AN OWNER'S MANUAL

As hands work their way through the day, lifting and manipulating, touching and holding, they are constantly exposed to challenges. Don't take them for granted: they deserve to be treated with care for the vital role they play in our daily lives. Protect them from harsh elements, exercise them for peak performance, relax them as a respite from work, and pamper them as a reward for the work they do.

Just as it is important to warm up before embarking on an exercise routine, the hands too will benefit from a few warm-up exercises to prepare them for their day's work. A quick routine of stretches in the morning will help improve performance and prevent injury. Repeat these exercises at intervals during the day to ease fatigue and maintain flexibility.

CREATE YOUR OWN HAND SPA

Hands appreciate pampering, from slathering with hand lotion, to having a professional manicure or hand-reflexology session. So create your own hand spa, where you can indulge your hands whenever they feel in need. Soak tired hands in a bowl of warm water, get the circulation going by rubbing with a loofah, rub them dry with a warm, soft towel, then apply a generous helping of hand lotion. Wear cotton gloves in bed to ensure that the hand lotion has maximum impact. A warm paraffin-wax bath is a luxurious addition to your hand spa, providing even more relaxing, moisturizing, and warming benefits.

SKIN CARE

For many individuals, the work they do challenges the skin on the hands. If the job includes frequent hand-washing, especially with hot water and harsh soap — as, for example, in a hospital setting — protective oils in the skin are lost, leading to dry skin and chapping. The hands of outdoor workers come in for particularly heavy use and need extra care to avoid problems. In general, use cool water and mild soap to wash the hands, followed by the use of hand lotion. Generously moisturize the hands at night before going to bed.

Don't use your hand as a hammer: while you may never have done this, we can assure you that others have.

HAND-CARE DOS AND DON'TS

- Wearing gloves can prevent many hand injuries, so wear them whenever necessary. Wear gloves appropriate to the activity: strong, protective gloves for gardening; cloth-lined vinyl gloves when washing dishes or using cleaning compounds; cotton gloves when doing housework, to prevent the dryness caused by dust. And always wear gloves when out in cold weather.
- Be aware of safety in the kitchen, especially when using sharp knives. Grasping a bagel while cutting it, for example, results in some 100,000 visits to emergency rooms each year.
- When working in the garage or workshop, be cautious when using electric or hand tools.
- Help avoid injury by building hand awareness.

USING SELF-HELP TOOLS

Self-help hand reflexology techniques do not always reach deep areas, and not everyone has the strength or mobility to apply hand reflexology techniques, but using golf balls or other tools can provide an effective alternative. A golf ball is a good, inexpensive option, but you may prefer the softer surface of a rubber ball. Round and cylindrical rubber pet toys also make great tools.

You don't have to purchase the specialist reflexology self-help tools shown below. A generic rubber ball can work just as well.

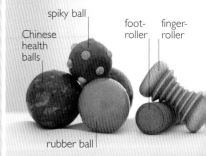

spiky ball

Chinese health balls

foot-roller

finger-roller

rubber ball

Using health balls

Health balls (*see below*) are typically made of metal or smooth, round polished rock, and they are meant to be used in pairs. Throughout China, Japan, and the rest of the Far East, where reflexology is common practice, health balls are a familiar sight in shops. Supplementing your hand-reflexology routines with the use of health balls several times a week can help to build flexibility in the hands, strengthen muscles in the reflex areas, and develop hand awareness. To use them, hold both balls in one hand and, using the digits of the same hand, move them in a clockwise or counter-clockwise direction. Then change hands and repeat. If you do not have access to health balls, try using two golf balls instead. However, you may find that the heavier weight of health balls makes them more suitable for the exercise.

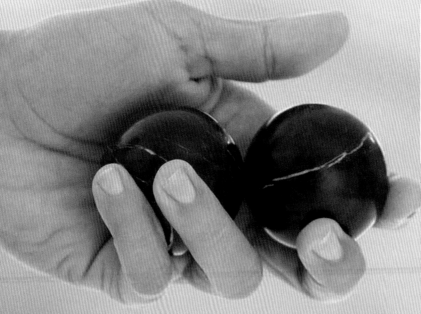

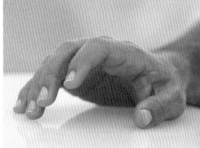

The action for moving health balls around the hand is similar to that of drumming the fingers on a flat surface (*see above*). Strike first with the little finger, then the other digits, in turn.

Cupping

Precision is not paramount in this technique. The rolling action is very effective for reaching several reflex areas on the palm at once. Before you start, remember that you should never use self-help tools on someone else; these exercises are for self-help only.

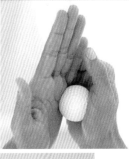

1 Cup the ball in the right hand, pressing with the fingers to create pressure and to keep the ball in place.

2 Now roll the ball around the left palm. Don't worry too much about where the pressure is applied. By rolling around the palm, you will cover a variety of reflex areas.

Pressing

This technique allows you to reach reflex areas located in the heels of both hands simultaneously. Increase the pressure by tightening your grip.

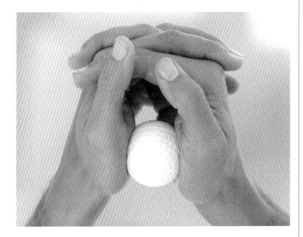

Interlace the fingers of both hands, trapping the ball between the heels of the hands. Roll the ball around, tightening or loosening the grasp to alter the pressure.

Gripping

Use this technique to work the reflex areas on and around the fingers and thumbs. Be careful not to overwork the areas by using too much pressure.

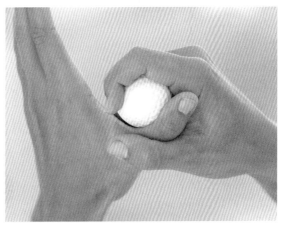

Hold the ball with the index and middle fingers of the right hand. Rest the ball on the left thumb, as shown, wrapping the right thumb around the top of the hand.

RELAXATION EXERCISES

The aim of these relaxation exercises is to provide the hands with a series of stretches to prepare them for work and to break up the habitual, limited patterns that are often followed during the day, leading to stress and injury in many cases. The exercises provide a particularly useful warm-up for those whose work involves the repetitive task of keyboarding.

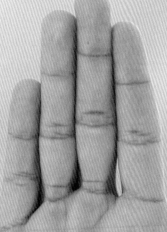

Tendon-glide exercises

These exercises help to prevent fatigue in the fingers and hands by working and strengthening under-used muscles.

1 Hold your hand upright with the fingers and thumb outstretched.

2 Leaving the thumb straight, curl your fingers in on themselves, making a hook.

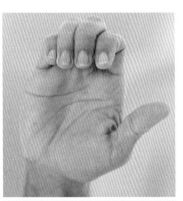

3 Still keeping your thumb straight, curl your fingers over and touch the palm with the fingertips.

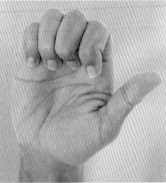

4 Curl the fingers and thumb into a fist and squeeze. Repeat several times.

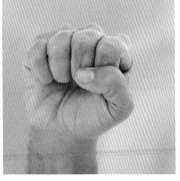

LEARNING TIP

Practice the tendon-glide exercises before work, repeating each one 3–5 times to start with, and gradually working up to 10 repetitions. Use the directional-movement stretches throughout the day to provide relaxation for the hands.

Directional-movement stretches

For those who regularly perform a repetitive task such as typing, it is important to break up habitual stress patterns. These exercises, known as directional-movement stretches, are particularly useful.

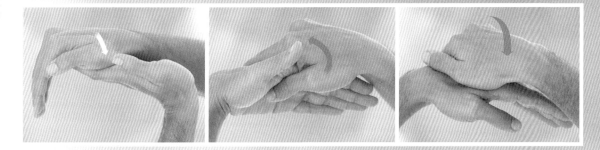

1 Position the left hand with the palm facing upward. Rest the right hand on the palm, with the heel at the base of the fingers. Press down with the fingers of the top hand. Hold for several seconds, then change hands and repeat.

2 Rest one hand on top of the other, with the fingers wrapped around the inner aspect of the hand. Press down with the fingers of the top hand, hold momentarily, then change hands and repeat.

3 Again resting one hand on top of the other, wrap the fingers around the outer aspect of the lower hand. Press down with the heel of the top hand, hold the position briefly, then change hands and repeat.

4 Finally, rest one hand on top of the other. Press down with the heel of the upper hand for a few seconds before changing hands and repeating the exercise.

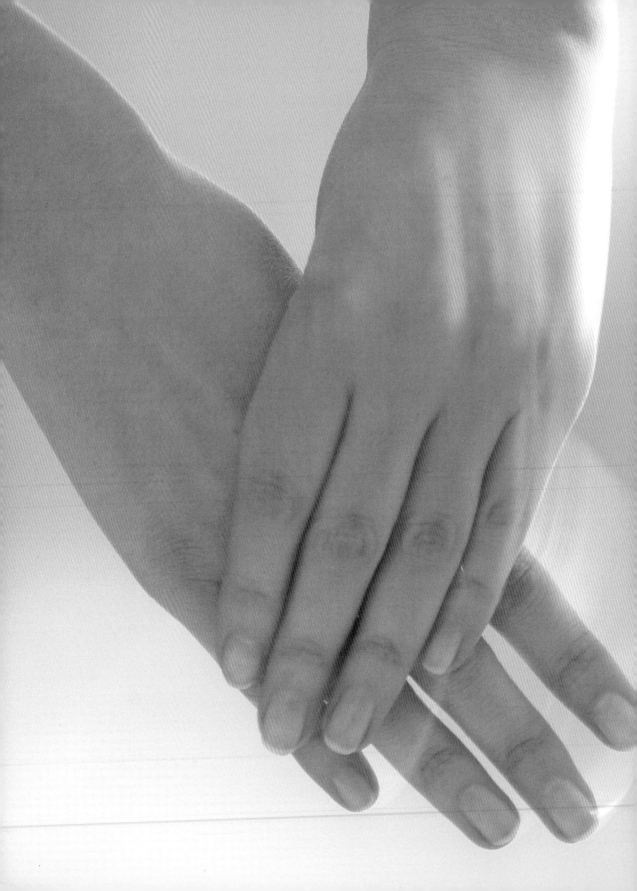

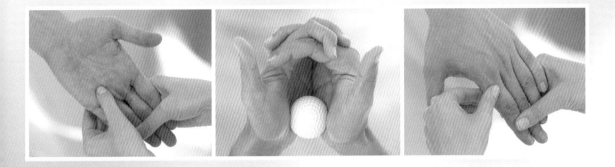

THE HAND-REFLEXOLOGY SESSION

The following section will show you how to improve your health and keep your hands happy. From a tutorial on the basic techniques to a series of step-by-step sequences, we take you through the essentials of giving a hand-reflexology session. It includes not only a complete hands-on reflexology sequence and a self-help sequence, but also an extra workout featuring self-help tools.

PREPARING FOR A REFLEXOLOGY SESSION

As you prepare for a hand-reflexology workout, it is essential to take all the steps necessary to create a pleasant experience for both you and your recipient. You will improve the chances of achieving the relaxation goals of your work if you apply some forethought about providing a comfortable setting, body positioning, and all the practical aspects of applying technique to hands.

GETTING READY

Step one in preparing for a reflexology session is to make sure that your fingernails are of an appropriate length. The nails of the working finger and thumb should not make contact at any time with the skin of the hand on which you are working. In general, when looking at your fingernails, your fingertip should protrude only very slightly beyond your nail. Take care, however, not to cut your nails too short.

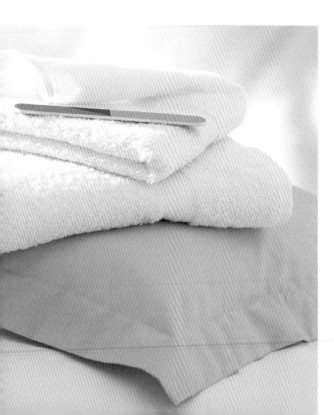

Look over your hands. If you see a cut or scratch in the skin, cover it with a dressing. You should always keep a supply nearby in case you need one for yourself or the recipient before you begin a session. The goal here is to avoid any risk of blood-to-blood contact.

You should always wash your hands before and after your reflexology sessions: this is a necessity since it assures the reflexology recipient of a pleasantly clean and hygienic session. It's a good habit to get into, even if you're just applying technique to yourself.

OPTIMUM POSITIONING

When preparing for a hand-reflexology session, you should remember that comfort is essential. Always aim to perform your reflexology work on a soft, but firm surface. This could comprise a pillow or a folded towel, whichever you prefer. Both are padded surfaces on which work can be done comfortably.

In an ideal situation, the recipient sits stretched back and relaxed in a recliner with a hand resting on a pillow or towel placed on the arm rest. The reflexologist sits alongside in another chair (preferably with wheels for easy repositioning). It is easiest if the reflexologist sits

Before starting your session, gather together any equipment you may need, such as pillow, towels, nail scissors or emery board, and hand lotion.

to the right-hand side of the recipient when applying work to the right hand and to the left-hand side of the client when applying work to the left hand. Reaching across the client to work on the opposite hand can be awkward and uncomfortable. Recipient and reflexologist may also sit face-to-face over a narrow table with the recipient's hand resting on a towel or pillow. Alternatively, you may sit side-by-side, with the recipient's hand placed on a folded towel or pillow resting on your knee.

OTHER ISSUES

When working with somebody's hands, consider yourself to be politely, yet firmly, in control of the hand to which you are applying technique. Be aware that working on another person's hands may be a little awkward at first. This is because of the perceptions about "hand-

To help tired hands relax, you might like to try some self-help aids such as a loofah or exfoliating mitt, rough towel, and vibrating massage wand.

holding" and the personal nature of touching someone else's hands. In order to proceed in a manner that is comfortable for both you and the recipient, you should aim to employ thoughtful "hand courtesy" before beginning the session.

Communication is key. Always tell the recipient when you are about to start or finish a reflexology session. Just before you begin a session, ask permission with a question such as "May I have your hand?" This serves as notification that the session is beginning. The phrase "I've finished — you may have your hand back" signals the end of a session. Should any interruption arise during the session, the same beginning and ending phrases may be used.

Maintaining physical contact during a reflexology session is also important. As you move from technique to technique, use the holding hand to maintain contact with the hand being worked. Such contact adds a smoothness and continuous level of comfort to the workout. In addition, it will be more convenient if the individual removes any rings, bracelet, or a watch that may interfere with your work. Have a bowl or basket available in which to place jewelry during the session.

BEGINNING THE SESSION

At the start of your work, ask the client if any part of the hand is injured or should be avoided. Older clients may complain of painful, enlarged, or arthritic finger joints. Approach conditions like this with caution.

Always begin and end your session with a series of desserts. This ensures some warm-up time for the hand, and provides a pleasant ending. Stay in touch with the individual as you apply techniques, bearing in mind that tastes vary. Some people favor a light touch applied to their hands while others like a vigorous workout. It's a good idea to ask the recipient what he or she prefers.

You should also make sure you work within the recipient's comfort zone by asking him or her how it feels. You could initiate the session by asking "will you tell me if the pressure is too much?" Bear in mind that there is a difference between "it hurts good" (which people really do say) and "it hurts."

A thorough hand reflexology workout may last 30–45 minutes. In the beginning, however, you might consider starting with shorter sessions. Mini-workouts are a good starting point for building hand strength. As your thumb and hands get stronger, you can build up to a full 45 minutes.

TARGETING HEALTH CONCERNS

After you've worked through the hand, it's time to consider other areas of emphasis: these are areas that need extra attention. To choose such areas, consider what it is you would like to achieve. If you have a specific health problem or hand disorder that needs addressing, turn to Chapter 5 and choose either Reflexology to Target Health Concerns (*see pages 122–139*) or Reflexology to Target Hand Concerns (*see pages 140–153*). Locate your specific health or hand concern in order to find helpful reflexology techniques. Alternatively, consult the reflexology charts (*see pages 16–19*). Apply a series of desserts again after working specific areas.

Now move on to the other hand, where you'll repeat the above. When you've finished your work with the second hand, it's time for a closing series of desserts.

KEY TO TECHNIQUE SYMBOLS	
Finger-walking	
Thumb-walking	
Hook & back-up	
Squeeze	
Pressure	
Traction, pulling, pushing, or side-to-side	
Rotation or rotation on a point	
Twist	
Palm-rocker	

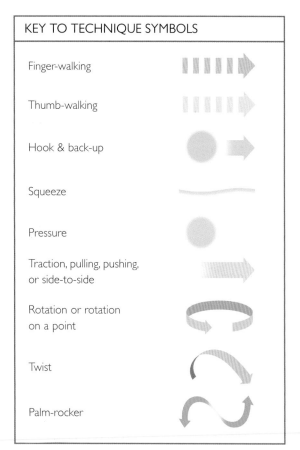

TIPS FOR AVOIDING TIREDNESS

TIME: Give yourself time to learn: just as when acquiring any skill, practice and time are needed.

POSITION: Make sure you have a comfortable working position that does not put unnecessary stresses and strains on your body.

TECHNIQUE: Review your technique application – done properly, your hands should not tire too easily.

STRENGTH: Practice self-help reflexology (see pages 86–101) to help build your strength.

DESSERTS: Take a tip from the professionals and break up your work with "desserts" (see pages 82–85), since these provide a chance for your working thumb or finger to have a rest.

CHANGE HANDS: Swap working hands regularly – if one thumb tires, adapt and apply technique with your other thumb.

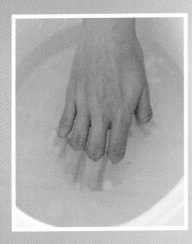

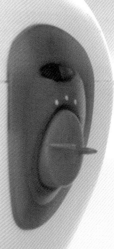

Soothe away aches and pains and give tired hands a treat by immersing them in the moisturizing warmth of a paraffin-wax bath.

RELAXING HANDS

Busy hands deserve a properly thought-out relaxation plan. Choose from the following ideas:

Sit quietly, resting your hands, perhaps in warm water.

Invest in a self-help tool such as an electric vibrating wand or a paraffin-wax bath.

Roll a foot-roller over your hand to provide general relaxation. Or, for an instant relaxation effect, rub vigorously with a loofah or coarse, exfoliating mitt.

Apply hands-on reflexology technique and desserts, targeting specific areas of concern.

Using a paraffin bath adds an extra, relaxing element to your reflexology session. Be sure to follow the manufacturer's instructions and, when you first start to use it, be aware of your response.

TECHNIQUES

In this section we describe four basic reflexology techniques: thumb-walking and finger-walking allow the application of pressure to a broad area of the hand, while the hook and back-up technique and rotating on a point both target reflex points deep in the fleshy parts of the hand. Practice these techniques on your own hand or forearm to help you build up your strength and skills.

Thumb-walking

The most efficient and effective technique in hand reflexology, thumb-walking applies a constant, steady pressure over the area being worked. As with any skill, it takes time to become proficient so practice on yourself till you perfect your technique. If your thumb becomes tired as you're learning, rest, change hands, or apply desserts (*see pages 82–85*).

LEARNING TIP

To find the proper angle of your thumb for thumb-walking, lay your hand down on a table. Note how the thumb rests on the table: the outer edge making contact with the table is the part of the thumb that should make contact with the hand being worked on. This angle makes the most of the leverage available from the four fingers.

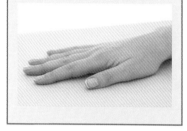

Practicing the technique

The basis for the thumb-walking technique is the bending and unbending of the first joint of the thumb. The goal is to take small "bites," creating a feeling of steady pressure as you inch forward.

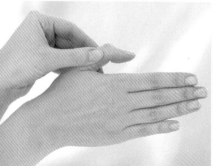

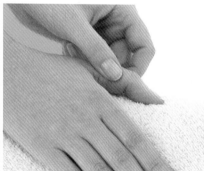

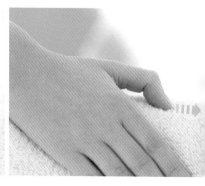

1 To practice the thumb action of this technique, hold the thumb below the first joint to prevent movement of the second joint. Now bend and straighten the first joint several times.

2 Still holding your thumb, position its outer edge on your leg. Bend and straighten the thumb several times, noting the pressure on your leg. Rock the thumb a little from the tip to the lower edge of the nail.

3 Remove the holding hand from your thumb and "walk" the thumb forward. Do not push it forward: bending and unbending are the sole means by which the thumb moves forward.

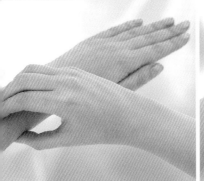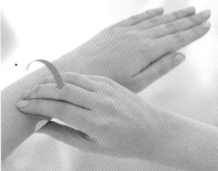

4 To practice using leverage, place the fingers and thumb of your right hand on your forearm. Working together, these provide the leverage necessary to create pressure.

5 Lower the wrist of your working arm so that the thumb exerts pressure on the arm. This pressure is directed through the thumb, but actually results from the actions of the fingers, hand, and forearm.

6 Now bend and unbend your thumb, taking a little step forward with each "unbend." Continue practicing on your forearm until you produce a constant, steady pressure.

Applying the technique

Before thumb-walking on the palmar surface of the hand, first create a smooth, even surface on which to work. Stretch out the palm of the hand with the holding hand, as shown.

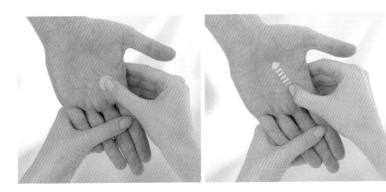

1 With the holding hand, stretch out the hand to be worked on. Place your thumb on the palm then drop your wrist to create leverage – this has the effect of exerting pressure with the thumb.

2 Keeping the hand in position, thumb-walk down the palm by bending and unbending the thumb. Reposition the thumb and thumb-walk down a different part of the hand.

COMMON MISTAKES

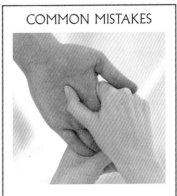

A frequent mistake when learning the thumb-walking technique is to overly bend the first joint of the thumb, resulting in stress to the thumb and possibly to the whole hand. It may also cause the thumb nail to dig into the skin. Another common error is to bend the second joint of the thumb instead of the first, again overworking the thumb and causing strain.

Finger-walking

Like the thumb-walking technique, finger-walking uses the bending and unbending of the first joint of the finger to "walk" over an area of the hand. The technique is well suited to working on the thinner skin on the top and sides of the hand. Multiple finger-walking feels good and has the advantage of working a broad area of the hand.

Practicing the technique

The "walking" motion of this technique is produced by a slight rocking action from the fingertip to the edge of the fingernail.

LEARNING TIP

Beginners often find that the finger "learns" this technique on its own, seemingly from the previously acquired skill of thumb-walking. As with thumb-walking, the finger must always move in a forward direction – never backward or sideways. The top of the hand is a good practice ground for finger-walking.

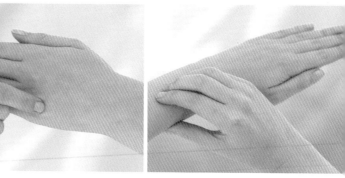

1 To practice the finger-walking movement, hold the index finger below the first knuckle to isolate the joint used in the technique. Practice bending and unbending the first joint of the index finger.

2 Using the same movement, "walk" the index finger up the back of the hand by bending and unbending the first joint, rocking the fingertip to the lower edge of the fingernail and back.

3 Use the finger and thumb in opposition to create leverage while finger-walking. To begin practicing, place the fingers on the forearm and the thumb underneath.

4 Raise the wrist as you hold on with the thumb and press the fingers into the forearm. Note the increased pressure that is now exerted by the fingers. Maintaining this pressure, "walk" the index finger forward, across the forearm.

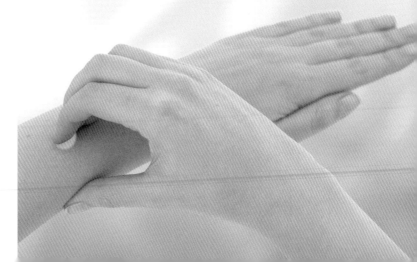

Applying the technique

As with thumb-walking, finger-walking requires the hand that is being worked on to be held steady by the holding hand, providing a stationary surface.

1 Hold the hand steady with the holding hand as shown. Place the tip of the index finger on the back of the hand and start finger-walking forward toward the wrist.

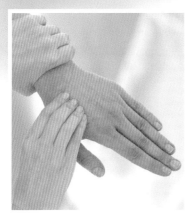

2 To practice multiple finger-walking, place the working fingers on top of the hand with the thumb resting at the wrist underneath. Now, bend and unbend the first joints of all four fingers as you "walk" them forward.

COMMON MISTAKES

Overbending the index finger is one of the most common mistakes when practicing the finger-walking technique. Keep your index finger parallel to the hand, bending and unbending the first joint as you inch forward. Other mistakes include moving your whole hand rather than just the first joint; digging the fingernail into the skin; and rolling the finger from side to side.

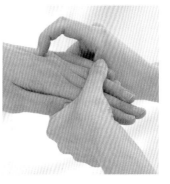

Hook & back-up

This technique is used to work a specific reflex point, rather than to cover a large area as in thumb-walking and finger-walking (*see pages 54–57*). It is a relatively stationary technique, with the working finger making only very small movements.

Practicing the technique

Leverage is important in applying deeper pressure – here, the palm of your hand provides a backstop for the pressure being applied by the index finger. It is important that deep pressure is applied to the correct area: sensitivity is an indicator that you're on the right spot.

1 Grasp the hand with the tip of the index finger resting at the center of the thumb. Bend the finger to press into the thumb, then pull back to exert pressure. Brace the thumb against the thumb of the working hand.

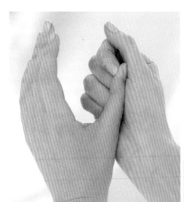

2 To practice on the palm of the hand, place the index finger as shown. Bend the finger, pressing into the hand, then pull back. Note how the thumb serves as a backstop.

Applying the technique

Keep the hand steady with the holding hand as the technique is applied. If the fingers curl forward impeding access, hold them back.

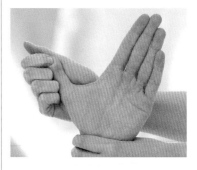

1 Place the tip of the index finger in the center of the thumb, curl the finger, and exert pressure on the PITUITARY reflex area.

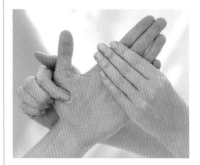

2 Move the tip of your index finger to the ADRENAL GLAND reflex area in the fleshy part of the thumb, and exert pressure.

Rotating on a point

This technique is used to work the bonier parts of the wrist. The index finger pinpoints the reflex area, while the holding hand moves the recipient's hand first in a clockwise and then in a counter-clockwise direction.

2 Reposition your index finger on the wrist, in the hollow at the base of the ring finger, and repeat the technique, rotating the hand first in a clockwise and then in a counter-clockwise direction.

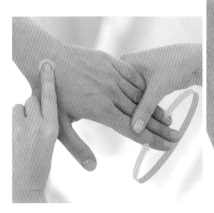

1 Rest the tip of your index finger on the top of the wrist, in the hollow at the base of the index finger, as shown. Grasp the fingers with your holding hand, as shown, and move the hand first in a clockwise and then in a counter-clockwise direction.

LEARNING TIP

Keep a relaxed but firm grip on the recipient's fingers with the holding hand, taking care not to pinch the fingers together. As you rotate the hand, imagine you're drawing a circle in the air with the tips of the fingers.

HAND DESSERTS

The desserts described on the following pages are techniques that relax the hand through stretch and movement, as well as exploring its flexibility and range of movement. They may serve as a soothing interlude aimed solely at relaxation; or they can be used as part of a session — at the beginning and end, and as a transition between steps in a sequence. Be careful not to over-apply hand desserts, moving the finger joints more than they can comfortably absorb. If relaxation is the goal of the session, keep your actions slow and easy.

1 To apply the hand-stretcher technique, grasp the hand as shown (*see left*) and turn both wrists outward, pressing up on the palm with your fingers as you do so.

Hand-stretcher

This dessert relaxes the body of the hand, helping to break up stress patterns that have been set up during the day. Proceed gradually and gently as you move the hand, pausing between the upward and downward stretches.

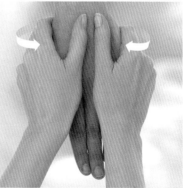

2 Now turn your wrists inward as you press the top of the hand with your palms. Repeat these two actions alternately several times.

Palm-rocker

This dessert is most effective when applied rhythmically, relaxing the hand as well as preparing it for further work. Movement is created between the long bones of the hand by moving them back and forth alternately. Be careful not to over-apply this dessert.

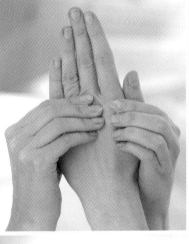

2 Reverse the action, pushing with the left hand and pulling with the right. Alternate the two movements several times.

1 Clasp the hand as shown, with the flats of the fingers along the long bone of the index finger. Push toward the fingers with the right hand while you pull toward the wrist with the left.

Palm-mover

This dessert promotes flexibility and relaxation of the whole hand by gently moving the long bones. Repeat the dessert several times on the long bone of each finger.

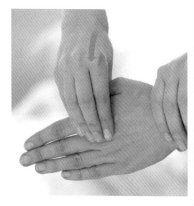

1 Press gently along the long bone of the index finger, while pulling up with the thumb to create counter-movement. Repeat on the long bone of the middle finger.

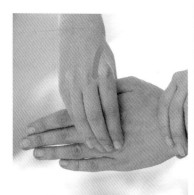

2 Move on to the long bone of the ring finger, pressing with the fingers and pulling up with the thumb. Repeat the sequence on the long bone of the little finger.

Palm counter-mover

Using a movement in counter-direction to that of the palm-mover, this technique provides another way of creating movement between the long bones of the hand. In this case, the flat of the thumb rests on top of the hand, providing padding for the bony surface as it is pushed downward, while the fingers pull up from below.

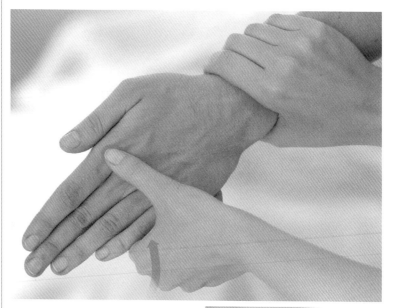

1 Rest your working thumb on the knuckle of the index finger. Push downward with the thumb and pull up with the working hand to turn the outside of the hand upward. Release and repeat several times.

LEARNING TIP

Practice this technique on your own hand to see how it feels. Press down on the knuckle of the index finger and hold for several seconds. Repeat on each knuckle of both hands, comparing tension levels.

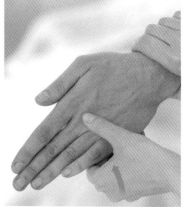

2 Moving the thumb to each of the knuckles in turn, repeat the movement several times, pushing down with the thumb and pulling up with the fingers.

Finger side-to-side

In this hand-dessert technique, the finger joints are moved in a way that is different from normal. While the holding hand keeps the finger steady and the upper joints static, the working hand creates a slight side-to-side movement at the joint that is being worked on.

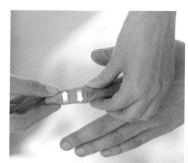

1 To work on the index finger, hold it static at the middle joint with the holding hand. Grasp the fingertip between the index finger and thumb and move the first joint from side to side.

LEARNING TIP

Increase movement in the finger joint gradually, always keeping within the recipient's comfort zone. Maintain a smooth, steady, rhythmic movement to create the greatest relaxation.

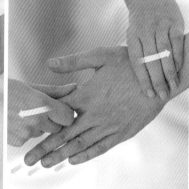

2 Repeat the side-to-side movement of the index finger several times, then move on and apply to each digit in turn.

Finger-pull

This technique provides an easy way to relax the whole hand. The gentle pull loosens the finger joints, relieving the compression that can occur as a result of routine tasks such as keyboarding.

LEARNING TIP

Wrap your fingers around the digit being worked, making full contact; a firm, even pressure creates the most relaxing effect. As you pull the finger, remember to create a counter-pull with the holding hand.

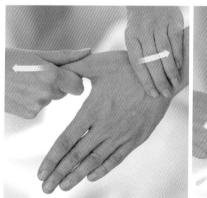

1 Grip the wrist with the holding hand. Grasp the thumb and pull it slowly and steadily toward you while pulling gently in the opposite direction with the holding hand.

2 Continue gripping the wrist with the holding hand and repeat the pulling action on the index finger, then on each of the other fingers and thumb in turn.

Walk-down / pull-against

This technique applies both pressure and stretch to encourage flexibility of the fingers. Bending the finger slightly beyond its normal range of movement enhances the digit's mobility.

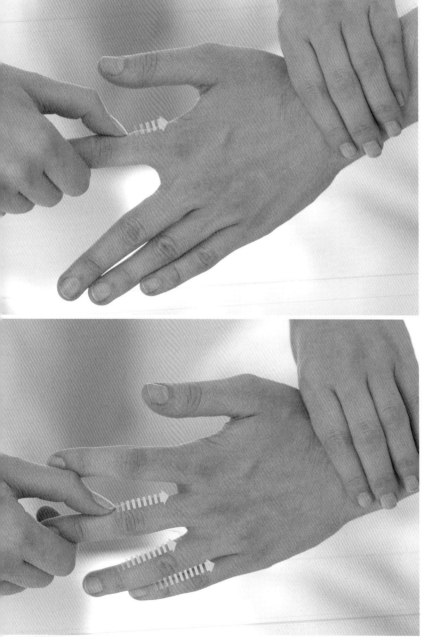

LEARNING TIP
The walk-down/pull-against technique is best applied with leverage for the walking thumb. Drop your wrist to create leverage, allowing your fingertips to work against the thumb tip.

1 Use the holding hand to grasp the wrist of the hand to be worked. Then position the working thumb and fingers (*see left*). Now thumb-walk down the side of the finger, while stretching the inside of the finger. Make several passes.

2 Move on to the middle finger and thumb-walk down the side of the finger while stretching the inside edge. Repeat the sequence on each digit. Focus particularly on the joints.

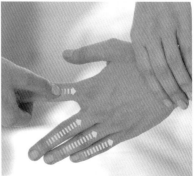

3 Once you've walked down the sides of the fingers, walk down the topside of each finger.

The squeeze

This is a simple, yet effective, technique that relaxes the whole hand from the fingertips to the wrist. Although the pictures below show the technique being applied to the whole hand, it can be used on the fingers individually, one at a time. Use a firm but gentle grasp when applying this hand dessert.

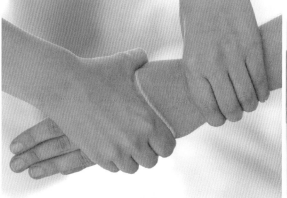

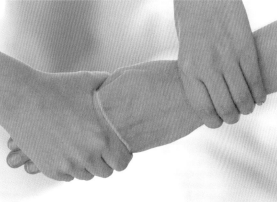

1 Using the holding hand, grasp the wrist to hold the hand steady. Now wrap your working hand around the base of the hand, near the wrist and gently, but firmly, squeeze the hand.

2 Reposition your working hand, now grasping the hand around the area of the knuckles. Again firmly apply pressure, squeezing the hand. Be careful not to squeeze the fingers together too hard.

LEARNING TIP

The squeeze is most effective when the whole surface of the working palm makes contact with the whole surface of the hand being worked.

3 Now reposition your working hand around the fingertips. Press gently, always staying within the recipient's comfort zone.

STEP 1

Working the fingers and the thumb

The areas worked in this sequence – the brain, pituitary, thyroid, and parathyroid – control many of the body's vital functions. As you work through the sequence, you'll be relaxing, stimulating, and enhancing the functioning of those organs as well as producing an overall respite from stress as the muscles relax. This, in turn, has a beneficial effect on the homeostatic balance of the body.

DESSERTS   Hand-stretcher (*p. 60*) • Palm-rocker (*p. 61*) • Palm-mover (*p. 62*) Palm counter-mover (*p. 62*) • Finger side-to-side (*p. 63*) Finger-pull (*p. 63*) • Walk-down/pull-against (*p. 64*)

AREAS WORKED

Head, Brain — Pituitary — Sinus

Neck

Thyroid, Para-thyroid

1 To work the PITUITARY reflex area, hold the hand steady and rest the thumb against the working hand, Press the reflex area repeatedly with the index finger.

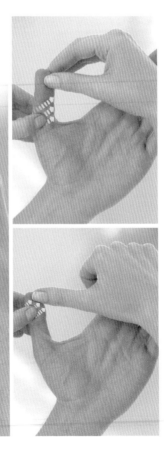

2 Reposition the holding hand and use the thumb-walking technique to apply a succession of passes across the thumb. Begin at the base of the thumb to work the NECK, THYROID, and PARATHYROID reflex areas.

3 Next, make a series of passes around the upper segment of the thumb, to work the HEAD, SINUS, and BRAIN reflex areas.

4 Straighten the hand, then thumb-walk across the NECK, HEAD, SINUS, and BRAIN reflex areas of the index finger. Repeat on the other fingers.

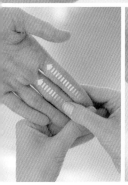

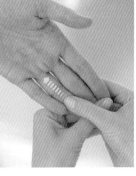

5 Now thumb-walk down the index finger and then the middle finger.

6 Go on to the ring finger and thumb-walk throughout the NECK, HEAD, SINUS, and BRAIN reflex areas.

7 Change hands and complete the coverage by thumb-walking down the little finger.

DESSERTS   Finger-pull (p. 63) • Walk-down/pull-against (p. 64)
Palm-rocker (p. 61)

HAND ORIENTATION

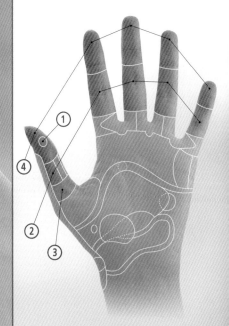

LEFT HAND

By working reflex areas on the fingers and thumb, this sequence targets structures in the head and neck.

The first segment of the thumb reflects the left half of the head, including all layers – from the surface of the skin to the deepest recesses of the brain. The PITUITARY GLAND ① is represented in the center of the first segment. Reflex areas of the thumb's second segment correspond to the NECK ② and THYROID and PARATHYROID GLANDS ③. The first segment of each finger represents a portion of the HEAD, BRAIN, and SINUSES ④. The next segment and half of the third segment relate to the base of the NECK. The reflex areas of the right hand mirror those of the left hand.

STEP 2

Working the thumb and webbing

This sequence works on reflex areas corresponding to the adrenal glands, the kidneys, and part of the stomach, relaxing, stimulating, and enhancing the functioning of those parts of the body. It also contributes to a general relaxation response by impacting on the blood and nerve supply. The hands themselves benefit from general relaxation and from the experiences of pressure and movement, both of which are important for maintaining their functions.

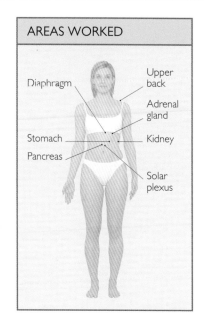

AREAS WORKED

Diaphragm
Upper back
Adrenal gland
Stomach
Kidney
Pancreas
Solar plexus

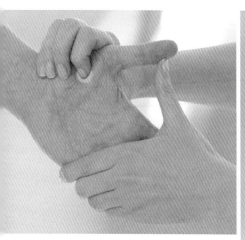

1 Holding the recipient's thumb and fingers as shown, rest the tip of your index finger on the ADRENAL GLAND reflex area, which is located in the fleshy palm at the midpoint of the long bone below the thumb. Exert pressure with the fingertip. A reaction of sensitivity will indicate that you've found the reflex area. Press repeatedly.

2 Reposition and begin a series of thumb-walking passes through the PANCREAS and STOMACH reflex areas on the heel of the thumb.

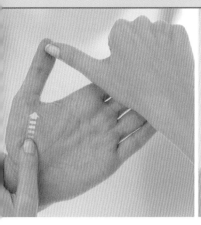

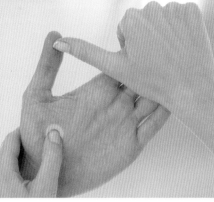

3 Reposition your thumb in the webbing of the hand and work the SOLAR PLEXUS, UPPER BACK and KIDNEY reflex areas with successive thumb-walking passes.

4 To work the KIDNEY reflex area more thoroughly, place your thumb and fingertips on opposite sides of the hand. Press into the reflex area on the webbing, holding for several seconds.

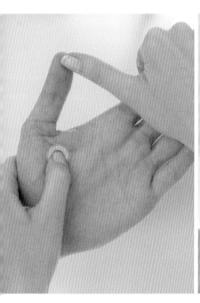

5 Reposition the thumb and fingertips in various parts of the webbing to press and work the DIAPHRAGM and UPPER BACK reflex areas.

6 Hold the hand upright. Link your hands and thumb-walk with both thumbs up the webbing. Reposition your thumbs and thumb-walk through another portion of the webbing.

DESSERTS   Finger-pull (p. 63) • Hand-stretcher (p. 60) • Palm-rocker (p. 61)

HAND ORIENTATION

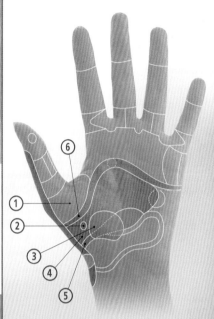

LEFT HAND

Working the reflex areas in the thumb, webbing, and fleshy palm of the hand targets a number of major organs as well as the upper back.

The palm below the thumb reflects the UPPER BACK (1) from neck to waist and from spine to shoulder blades. Also reflected in this area are certain vital organs: the ADRENAL GLAND (2), KIDNEY (3), portions of the STOMACH (4), and the PANCREAS (5). The DIAPHRAGM reflex area runs in a narrow band across the palm (6).

The reflex areas of the left webbing and palm differ from those of the right hand just as the left and right sides of the body do not exactly mirror each other. The stomach and pancreas lie primarily on the left side with the liver on the right. Matching organs such as the two kidneys and adrenal glands, however, are represented on each side.

STEP 3

Working the upper palm

This sequence works reflex areas that relate to the upper body, including the heart and lungs, which are responsible for blood and oxygen flow. As well as enhancing the function of these vital organs, the sequence also works on reflex areas of the musculoskeletal structure of the upper body, helping to relax the shoulders and the upper back. The sequence is completed by working the webbing between the fingers, which corresponds with the reflex areas for the eyes, inner ears, and ears.

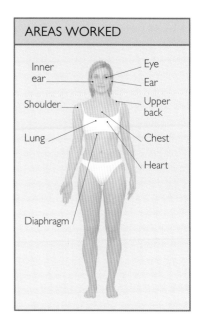

AREAS WORKED

Inner ear
Eye
Ear
Shoulder
Upper back
Lung
Chest
Heart
Diaphragm

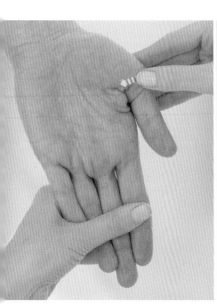

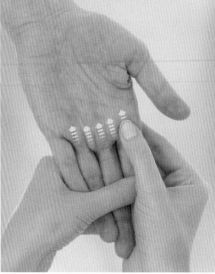

1 Hold the recipient's hand in place with the holding hand and thumb-walk across the base of the thumb to work the HEART reflex area, making several passes.

2 Working from the base of the fingers toward the DIAPHRAGM reflex area, thumb-walk through the CHEST, LUNG, and UPPER BACK reflex areas in successive passes.

3 Change hands so that the right hand holds the fingers steady and the left hand applies the thumb-walking technique. Thumb-walk across the SHOULDER reflex area, making several passes and contouring around the bone.

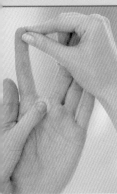
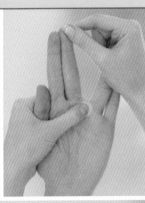
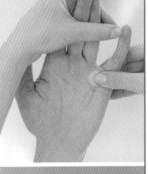

HAND ORIENTATION

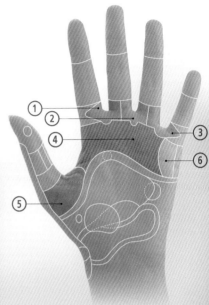

4 Hold the index and middle fingers apart with the holding hand. Place the thumb and fingertips on either side of the webbing and press gently several times on the EYE reflex area.

5 Move on to work the INNER EAR reflex area, gently pinching the webbing several times.

6 Change hands and work the EAR reflex area, pinching the webbing gently several times with the right hand.

7 Holding the recipient's hand upright as shown, interlace your fingers and continue working on the EYE, INNER EAR, and EAR reflex areas in the webbing between the fingers. Thumb-walk with one thumb on either side of the webbing.

LEFT HAND

Working the upper palm targets three groups of reflex areas: the eyes and ears; the chest, lungs, and heart; and the shoulders and upper back.

The EYE ①, INNER EAR ②, and EAR ③ reflex areas are located in the webbing between the fingers. These overlap with reflex areas corresponding to the base of the neck and the tops of the shoulders as well as the blood and nerve supply to the eyes and ears. The CHEST, LUNG, and UPPER BACK ④ reflex area is a band across the top of the palm. The HEART ⑤ reflex area is located around the base of the thumb and the SHOULDER ⑥ reflex area is at the base of the little finger.

The reflex areas on the left hand mirror those on the right, with the left hand relating to the left side of the body and the right hand corresponding to the right.

DESSERTS Palm-rocker (p. 61) • Palm-mover (p. 62) • Palm counter-mover (p. 62)

STEP 4
Working the center and heel of the palm

The reflex areas worked in this sequence reflect organs responsible for digestion, such as the stomach, gall bladder, liver, small intestine, and colon. This sequence also includes reflex areas representing the upper and lower back. The arm reflex area, which lies in the fleshy outer edge of the hand below the little finger, is also included. Work on the center and heel of the palm results in relaxation of the back and improvement in the functioning of the digestive process as the relaxation response impacts on their nerve and blood supply.

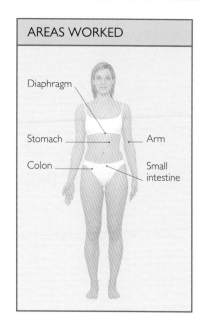

AREAS WORKED

Diaphragm

Stomach

Colon

Arm

Small intestine

1 To access the STOMACH reflex area, straighten the hand by clasping the fingers with the holding hand. Beginning at the DIAPHRAGM reflex area, apply a series of thumb-walking passes with the right thumb throughout the STOMACH reflex area.

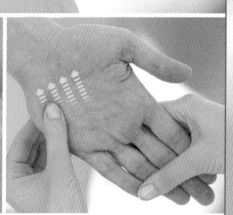

2 Change hands and hold the fingers back with your right hand while you continue thumb-walking through the STOMACH reflex area with the left thumb.

3 To work the ARM reflex, press the fleshy outer edge of the hand between the thumb and finger. Reposition and continue up the hand.

4 To work the COLON and SMALL INTESTINE reflex areas, hold the hand steady with your right hand and use your left thumb to make a series of thumb-walking passes.

DESSERTS   Palm-rocker (p. 61) • Hand-stretcher (p. 60) • Finger-pull (p. 63)

HAND ORIENTATION

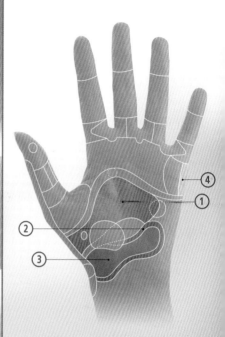

LEFT HAND

Working reflex areas in the center and heel of the palm targets mostly reflex areas relating to the digestive organs.

On the left hand is represented the portion of the digestive organs on the left side of the body. The STOMACH ① reflex area spans the palm. The COLON ② reflex area runs across the heel of the hand bordering the SMALL INTESTINE ③ area. The ARM ④ reflex area is located in the fleshy pad of the outer hand just below the little finger.

In addition, while not noted on many reflexology charts, this area also includes muscles and bones of the upper back and hip/lower back. Usually the reflex areas on the left and right hands mirror one another exactly. However, the stomach and spleen appear only on the left hand. The liver and gall bladder are represented on the right hand.

STEP 5

Working the tops of the fingers and the side of the thumb

In this sequence you work reflex areas that correspond to the spine (on the side of the thumb) and the head, neck, sinuses, teeth, gums, and jaw (on the fingers). The resulting relaxation improves the functioning of those body parts and their blood and nerve supply. To target a specific body part, pause for a few seconds and thumb-walk through the reflex area repeatedly. Work in this sequence also relaxes the fingers themselves, easing the discomfort of tired hands.

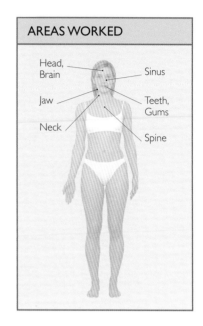

AREAS WORKED

Head, Brain — Sinus — Jaw — Teeth, Gums — Neck — Spine

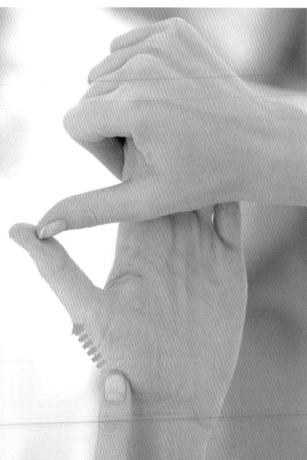

1 To work the SPINE reflex area, hold the hand steady and thumb-walk up the bony edge of the thumb, starting at the TAILBONE reflex area. Make several passes.

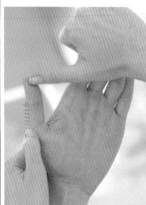

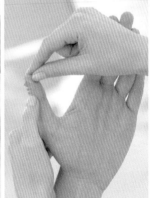

2 Continue thumb-walking through the SPINE reflex area, making several passes. Here the midback area is being worked.

3 Still holding the hand steady with the right hand, thumb-walk through the NECK reflex area of the spine with the left thumb.

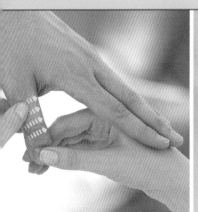 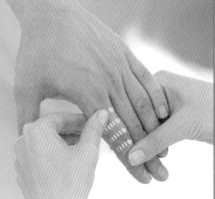

HAND ORIENTATION

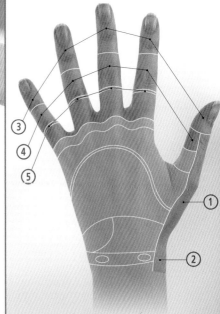

4 Change the position of the holding hand, resting the fingers on the back of the hand and holding the thumb stable to work the HEAD, BRAIN, SINUS, NECK, TEETH, GUMS, and JAW reflex areas. Thumb-walk around the thumb, making several, successive passes.

5 Now holding the fingers in place with the right hand, walk the left thumb around the index finger in successive passes. After you've covered the whole index finger in this way, go back and make successive passes over the first joint of the index finger. Move on to the second joint and repeat.

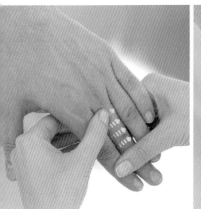 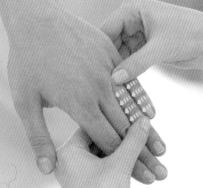

6 On the middle finger, work the next portion of the HEAD, BRAIN, SINUS, NECK, TEETH, GUMS, and JAW reflex areas in a series of passes.

7 Change hands to work the HEAD, BRAIN, SINUS, NECK, TEETH, GUMS, and JAW reflex areas on the ring finger before moving on to repeat the sequence on the little finger.

DESSERTS   Finger-pull (p. 63) • Hand-stretcher (p. 60)
Walk-down/pull-against (p. 64)

LEFT HAND

Working these areas targets the spine and the anatomical structures of the face and head.

On the left hand is represented the portion of these organs on the left side of the body. Replicating the way the spine runs down the back, the reflex area for the SPINE ① runs down the side of the thumb, with the TAILBONE area ② at the bottom near the wrist. The areas representing the HEAD, BRAIN, and SINUS ③ all occupy the same reflex area, which runs from the tip to the first joint on each of the five digits. Underneath this – again on each of the five digits – is the reflex area for the NECK ④. Finally the reflex area for the TEETH, GUM, and the JAW ⑤ is a very narrow band at the second joint on each finger.

The reflex areas on the right and left hand mirror one another perfectly.

STEP 6

Working the top of the hand

Working the reflex areas in this sequence relaxes and eases pain in parts of the musculoskeletal system, including the back and legs. Working the reflex areas on the top of the hand also stimulates and enhances functions such as heart action, respiration, lactation, and reproduction. The relaxation response is augmented as work on these reflex areas breaks up patterns of stress throughout the body. The work in this sequence also relaxes the hand itself, protecting it from overuse and injury, as well as improving its capabilities.

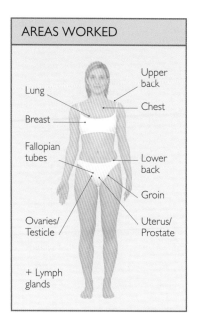

AREAS WORKED

Lung
Upper back
Chest
Breast
Fallopian tubes
Lower back
Groin
Ovaries/ Testicle
Uterus/ Prostate
+ Lymph glands

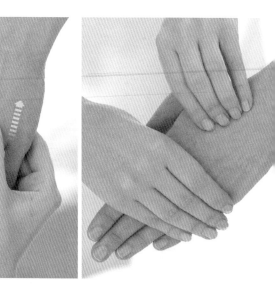

1 Steadying the hand with your right hand as shown above, work the LUNG, CHEST, BREAST, and UPPER BACK reflex areas by thumb-walking down the long bones (*see page 39*) around the webbing between the thumb and index finger. Make several passes.

2 Change hands to work the next part of these reflex areas. With the right thumb, thumb-walk between the long bones, making a series of passes down the top of the hand. Walk down the long bones to where they create a v-shaped indentation.

3 Reposition your holding hand to steady the recipient's hand as you use all four fingers to finger-walk across the KNEE, HIP, DIGESTIVE, and LOWER BACK reflex areas. Repeat several times. Reposition your fingers and finger-walk through another part of the hand.

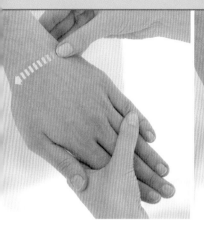

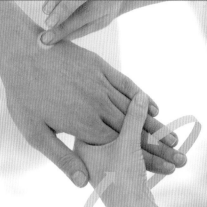

4 Still holding the hand with the right hand, walk the left thumb through the LYMPH GLANDS, FALLOPIAN TUBES, and GROIN reflex areas. Make a series of passes.

5 Pinpoint the OVARY / TESTICLE reflex area with the right index finger. Apply repeatedly the rotating-on-a-point technique (*see page 59*), clockwise then counter-clockwise.

HAND ORIENTATION

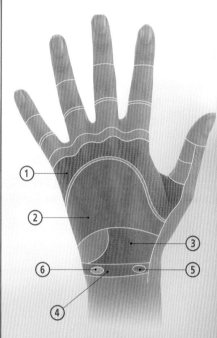

6 Change hands and pinpoint the UTERUS / PROSTATE reflex area. Rotate the hand repeatedly in a clockwise direction and then in a counter-clockwise direction as above.

LEFT HAND

The top of the hand contains reflex areas in wide bands. Close to the fingers is the reflex area for the UPPER BACK, LUNG, CHEST, and BREAST ①. (Note that all the reflex areas pass through the hand. Knuckles in the hand correspond to the shoulders, collar bones, and upper back.) Adjacent to this is another reflex areas for the UPPER BACK ② and, nearer the wrist, the reflex area for the LOWER BACK ③. In a narrow band near the wrist is the reflex area for the LYMPH GLANDS, FALLOPIAN TUBES, and GROIN ④. Within this is the reflex area for the TESTICLES/OVARIES ⑤ and for the PROSTATE/UTERUS ⑥.

The left hand mirrors the right hand: reflex areas on the right hand correspond to the right side of the body, while reflex areas on the left hand relate to the left.

DESSERTS   Finger-pull (p.63) • Walk-down/pull-against (p.64)
Palm-rocker (p.61).

STEP 7
Working the right hand

Now that you have worked through the full sequence on the left hand, it is time to move on to the right. An outline of the sequence for a right-hand workout is given on this and the following pages. Once you are familiar with how techniques are applied to each part of the hand, the summary will provide a useful reminder of the complete sequence.

DESSERTS

Before beginning the sequence, check the hand for cuts, bruises, and any other areas to be avoided during the workout

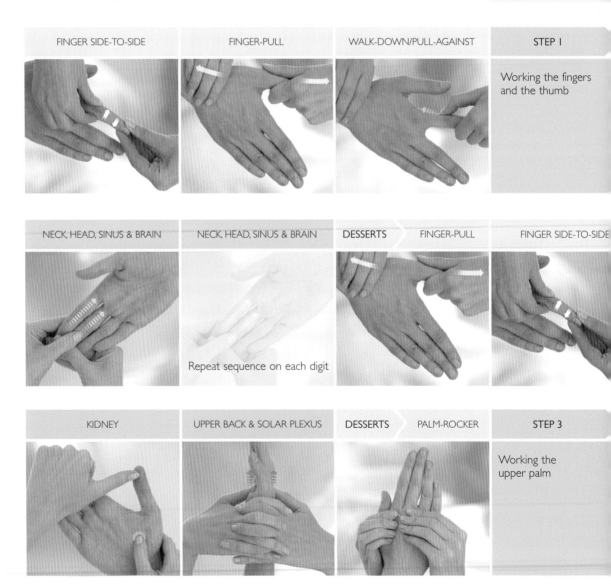

FINGER SIDE-TO-SIDE	FINGER-PULL	WALK-DOWN/PULL-AGAINST	**STEP I**
			Working the fingers and the thumb

NECK, HEAD, SINUS & BRAIN	NECK, HEAD, SINUS & BRAIN	**DESSERTS** FINGER-PULL	FINGER SIDE-TO-SIDE
	Repeat sequence on each digit		

KIDNEY	UPPER BACK & SOLAR PLEXUS	**DESSERTS** PALM-ROCKER	**STEP 3**
			Working the upper palm

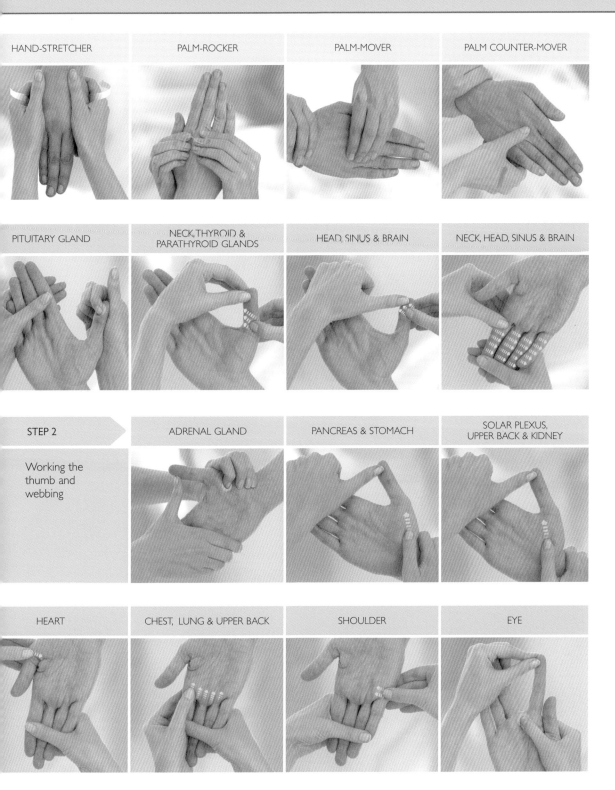

HAND-STRETCHER

PALM-ROCKER

PALM-MOVER

PALM COUNTER-MOVER

PITUITARY GLAND

NECK, THYROID & PARATHYROID GLANDS

HEAD, SINUS & BRAIN

NECK, HEAD, SINUS & BRAIN

STEP 2

Working the thumb and webbing

ADRENAL GLAND

PANCREAS & STOMACH

SOLAR PLEXUS, UPPER BACK & KIDNEY

HEART

CHEST, LUNG & UPPER BACK

SHOULDER

EYE

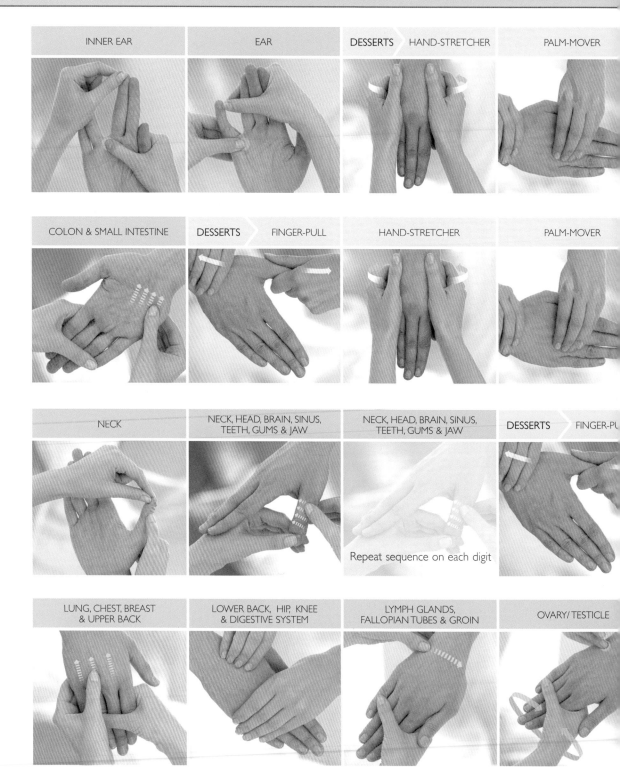

| INNER EAR | EAR | DESSERTS HAND-STRETCHER | PALM-MOVER |

| COLON & SMALL INTESTINE | DESSERTS FINGER-PULL | HAND-STRETCHER | PALM-MOVER |

| NECK | NECK, HEAD, BRAIN, SINUS, TEETH, GUMS & JAW | NECK, HEAD, BRAIN, SINUS, TEETH, GUMS & JAW | DESSERTS FINGER-PU |

Repeat sequence on each digit

| LUNG, CHEST, BREAST & UPPER BACK | LOWER BACK, HIP, KNEE & DIGESTIVE SYSTEM | LYMPH GLANDS, FALLOPIAN TUBES & GROIN | OVARY/ TESTICLE |

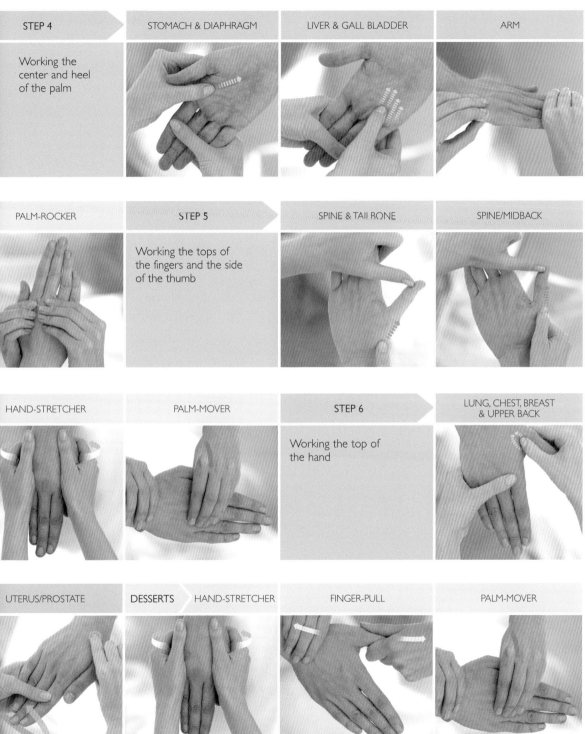

STEP 4	STOMACH & DIAPHRAGM	LIVER & GALL BLADDER	ARM
Working the center and heel of the palm			

PALM-ROCKER	STEP 5	SPINE & TAIL BONE	SPINE/MIDBACK
	Working the tops of the fingers and the side of the thumb		

HAND-STRETCHER	PALM-MOVER	STEP 6	LUNG, CHEST, BREAST & UPPER BACK
		Working the top of the hand	

UTERUS/PROSTATE	DESSERTS HAND-STRETCHER	FINGER-PULL	PALM-MOVER

SELF-HELP HAND DESSERTS

Dessert techniques feel good as they move the hand in directions not experienced every day. Use them singly, when you can snatch a moment, or use a series as a mini-vacation from routine. As you put this into practice and your body becomes more aware, you will respond more quickly to pain and learn how to manage stress levels.

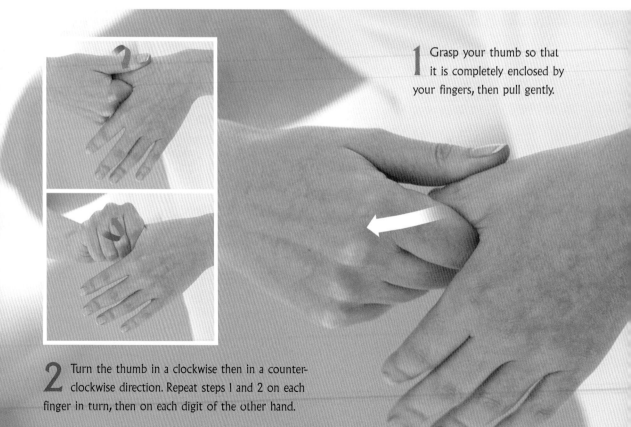

LEARNING TIP

The most effective desserts result from full contact with the hand. For example, when applying the finger-pull technique, the finger or thumb is completely enclosed by the hand. Understanding the structure of the hand will help you focus your efforts when applying desserts. Look at the anatomy maps on page 39 to help you visualize the joints.

Finger-pull

By creating traction, this gentle pull on the fingers loosens the joints and relieves compression. The technique relaxes the muscles of the fingers and helps to reset the tension level of the whole hand.

1 Grasp your thumb so that it is completely enclosed by your fingers, then pull gently.

2 Turn the thumb in a clockwise then in a counter-clockwise direction. Repeat steps 1 and 2 on each finger in turn, then on each digit of the other hand.

Finger side-to-side

The gentle rocking action of this dessert relaxes and loosens the finger joints, improving flexibility. Be sure to work within the joint's ability to absorb comfortably the side-to-side movement.

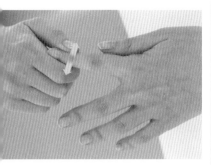

1 Grip your index finger between the opposite thumb and index finger to keep the top joint static. Push against the joint with the tip of your thumb then with the side of your index finger to create a side-to-side movement. Repeat several times.

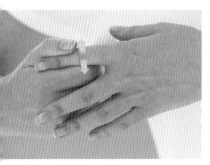

2 Repeat on the second joint then repeat steps 1 and 2 on each finger and on both thumbs.

Walk-down / pull-against

The goal of this dessert is to stretch the fingers in directions that are not commonly experienced during the day. As you thumb-walk down each finger to create stretch, you'll be applying pressure as well.

1 Rest the fingertips of your working hand on one side of your index finger and the thumb on the other. Thumb-walk down the outer aspect of the finger while stretching the inner side against your fingertips.

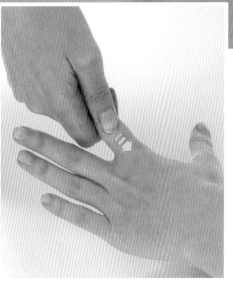

2 Change your grip on the index finger and thumb-walk down the upper aspect of the finger while stretching the finger back. Make several passes then repeat on each digit in turn.

Nail-buffing

This relaxing self-help dessert stimulates the circulation in the fingertips. Aim to perform the movement not only rapidly, but steadily, too. Once you've mastered the nail-buffing technique, it can be done discreetly anytime and anywhere.

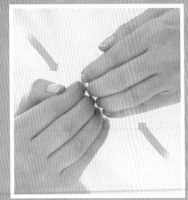

1   Rest both hands in front of you with the flats of the nails touching one another. Now rapidly and repetitively move the right hand in one direction, while simultaneously moving the left hand in the opposite direction. Without stopping, reverse the action, building up to a steady, rhythmic "buffing" motion.

Palm-mover

Using a movement that is similar to wringing the hands, the palm-mover technique induces feelings of relaxation by moving the long bones of the hands.

With the working hand, use the thumb to press gently along the long bone of each finger, while simultaneously pulling upward from the other side of the hand.

Palm counter-mover

The palm counter-mover is also effective for creating movement in the long bones of the hand, this time from the opposite direction to the palm-mover.

Use the working hand to press down on the knuckle of the index finger, while at the same time, using the thumb to twist the inside of the palm in an upward direction.

The squeeze

The squeeze uses gentle pressure that helps to relax the whole hand. Be careful not to squeeze too tightly, or it will have the opposite effect.

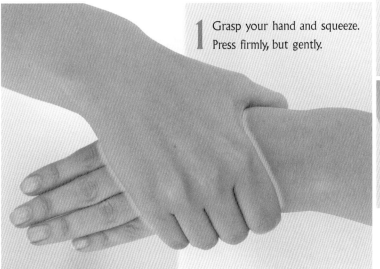

1 Grasp your hand and squeeze. Press firmly, but gently.

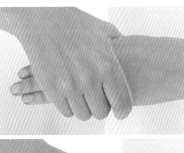

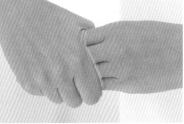

2 Reposition your hand and repeat as you squeeze successively closer to the fingertips.

STEP 1

Working the fingers and the thumb

The reflex areas worked in this sequence on the fingers and thumb include many that direct the body's activities, such as the brain, thyroid, parathyroid, and pituitary gland. In addition, you will work reflex areas corresponding to the head, brain, and sinuses; and jaw, teeth, and gums. At the end of the sequence, apply a series of desserts that are aimed at creating relaxation, such as the finger side-to-side and the walk-down/pull-against techniques.

DESSERTS   Finger-pull (p. 82) • Finger side-to-side (p.83) • Walk-down/
pull-against (p.83) • Nail-buffing (p.84) • Palm-mover (p.85)
Palm counter-mover (p.85) • The squeeze (p.85)

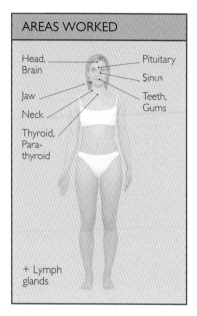

AREAS WORKED

Head, Brain — Pituitary
Jaw — Sinus
Neck — Teeth, Gums
Thyroid, Para-thyroid

+ Lymph glands

1 Rest the thumb against the thumb of the working hand. Press the tip of the index finger on the PITUITARY area in the center of the thumb. Press repeatedly, creating an on-off pressure.

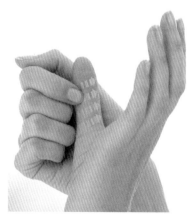

2 Holding the thumb steady against the knuckles of the working hand, use the finger-walking technique to make a series of passes across the thumb to work the following reflex areas: HEAD, BRAIN, SINUS; JAW, TEETH, GUMS; NECK, THYROID, and PARATHYROID.

3 Rest the hand, palm-up, on the working hand. Using the thumb-walking technique, make several passes across the entire index finger, working the HEAD, NECK, BRAIN, and SINUS areas. Concentrate particularly on the finger-joint areas.

HAND ORIENTATION

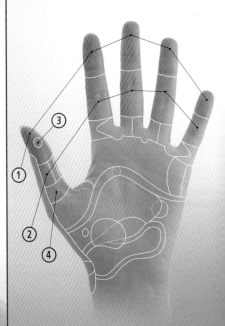

LEFT HAND

Working the reflex areas on the fingers and thumbs targets parts of the body around the head and neck.

At the tip of each finger is a reflex area that corresponds to the HEAD, BRAIN, and SINUSES ①. Below this, in the padded flesh between the first and second joints of each digit, is the reflex area for the NECK ②. The thumb, in addition to the reflex areas mentioned above, contains two other reflex areas: in the center of the fleshy pad at the top of the thumb is the PITUITARY GLAND reflex area ③; at its base is the reflex area for the THYROID and PARATHYROID GLANDS ④.

The reflex areas on the fingers and thumb of the left hand exactly mirror those on the right hand; the left hand relates to the left side of the body; the right hand to the right side of the body.

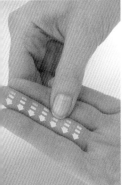

4 Thumb-walk over the same reflex areas on the middle finger.

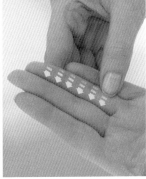

5 Move on to the ring finger and thumb-walk across the reflex areas as before.

6 Finally, apply the same technique to the reflex areas on the little finger.

DESSERTS   Finger side-to-side (p.83) • Walk-down/pull-against (p.83)

STEP 2

Working the thumb and webbing

Work in this sequence stimulates and enhances the functioning of the adrenal glands, pancreas, stomach, upper back, and kidneys — organs responsible for energy levels, digestion, and fluid processing. As you work on this fleshy part of the hand, take note of any nail marks that result from your application technique, and adjust it if necessary to lessen the impact.

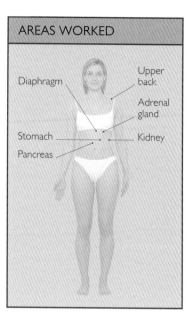

AREAS WORKED

Diaphragm

Upper back

Adrenal gland

Stomach

Kidney

Pancreas

1 Locate the ADRENAL GLAND reflex area by placing the tip of the index finger in the center of the fleshy palm, midway along the long bone below the thumb: sensitivity will indicate that you've found the reflex area. Press repeatedly.

2 Thumb-walk through the PANCREAS reflex area with the working thumb.

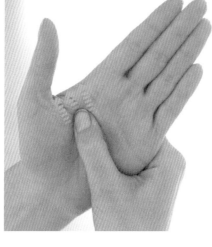

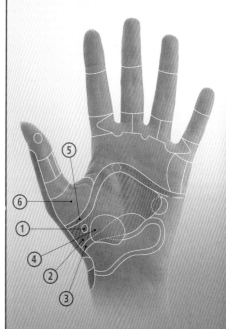

HAND ORIENTATION

3 Still using the thumb-walking technique, apply a series of passes through the STOMACH reflex area with the thumb of the working hand.

4 To work the DIAPHRAGM, UPPER BACK, and KIDNEY reflex areas, apply the thumb-walking technique in successive passes throughout the webbing and into the body of the hand.

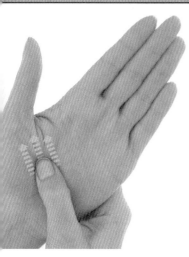

5 Finish by working more thoroughly on the KIDNEY reflex area: position the thumb and fingertips of the working hand in opposition to each other in the webbing. Press and release, moving around to find the most sensitive area. Press, adjusting pressure according to comfort level.

LEFT HAND

Working the reflex areas of the thumb and webbing focuses on a number of internal organs as well as on the upper back.

The reflex areas corresponding to the ADRENAL GLAND (1), STOMACH (2), PANCREAS (3), and KIDNEYS (4) are grouped together – just as those organs are grouped together in the body itself. Nearby, on the edge of the palm, above the DIAPHRAGM (5) reflex area, is the reflex area for the UPPER BACK (6).

With the exception of the reflex areas for the stomach and pancreas, the reflex areas on the left hand mirror those on the right; the left hand relates to the left side of the body and the right hand to the right side. The reflex area for the stomach is found only on the left hand; the pancreas reflex area is larger on the left hand.

DESSERTS   The squeeze (*p.85*) • Finger-pull (*p.82*)

STEP 3

Working the upper palm

Working the upper part of the palm targets reflex areas that correspond to three different parts of the upper body: the chest and lungs; the shoulders and upper back; and the eyes and ears. If you are aware that you hold stress in any of those areas, focus on the corresponding reflex areas as you work through the sequence here.

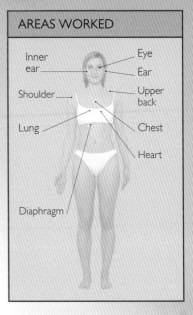

AREAS WORKED

Inner ear
Shoulder
Lung
Diaphragm
Eye
Ear
Upper back
Chest
Heart

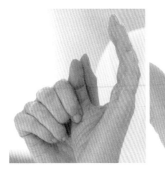

1 Using the tip of the index finger, finger-walk through the HEART reflex area in the direction of the arrow.

3 Move on to the SHOULDER reflex area and apply the thumb-walking technique in a series of passes.

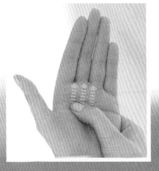

2 Starting at the DIAPHRAGM reflex area, thumb-walk in successive passes through all segments of the CHEST, LUNG, and UPPER BACK reflex areas.

4 To work the EYE reflex area, gently pinch the webbing with the thumb and index finger of the working hand. Repeat several times.

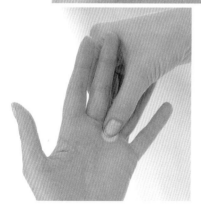

5 Work the INNER EAR reflex by gently pinching the webbing between the thumb and index finger, repeating several times.

6 Move on to the EAR reflex area and pinch the webbing gently between the thumb and index finger. Press repeatedly.

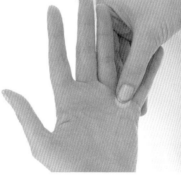

DESSERTS Palm-mover (p.85) • Palm counter-mover (p.85)

HAND ORIENTATION

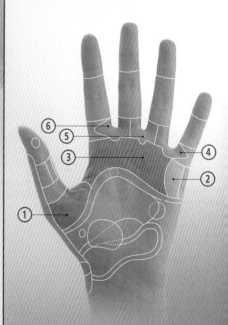

LEFT HAND

Working on the upper palm targets three groups of reflexes: eyes and ears; chest, lungs, and heart; and shoulders and upper back.

The HEART ① reflex area is located at the base of the thumb and that of the SHOULDER ② at the base of the little finger. The reflex area for the CHEST, LUNG, and UPPER BACK ③ is located in a band across the top of the palm. The EAR ④, INNER EAR ⑤, and EYE ⑥ reflex areas are located in the webbing between fingers.

The reflex areas on the left hand mirror those on the right; the left hand relates to the left side of the body and the right hand to the right side of the body. Note that all the reflex areas pass through the hand. Knuckles in the hand correspond to the shoulders, collar bones, and upper back.

STEP 4

Working the center and heel of the palm

The reflex areas worked here correspond to the stomach, colon, and small intestines. Also included in this part of the hand, which spans the fleshy outer edge below the little finger, is part of the upper back reflex area and the arm reflex area. As you thumb-walk through the fleshy palm be careful not to dig your nail into the skin.

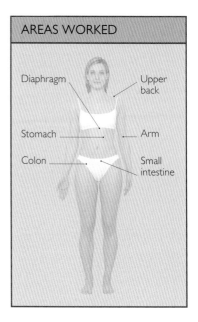

AREAS WORKED

Diaphragm
Upper back
Stomach
Arm
Colon
Small intestine

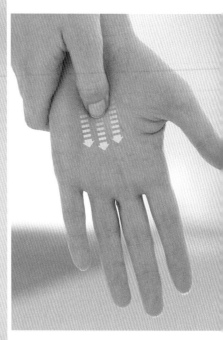

1 Thumb-walk through the STOMACH reflex area, ending in the DIAPHRAGM area. You will also be working part of the UPPER BACK.

2 Continue making a series of thumb-walking passes with the right thumb through the STOMACH and UPPER BACK reflex area.

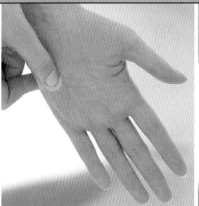

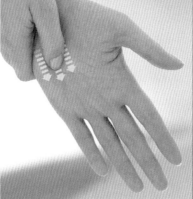

3 Move on to the ARM reflex, pressing the fleshy outer part of the hand between the thumb and index finger of the working hand. Continue up the hand.

4 To work the COLON and SMALL INTESTINE reflex, use your right thumb to make a series of thumb-walking passes through all segments of the reflex area.

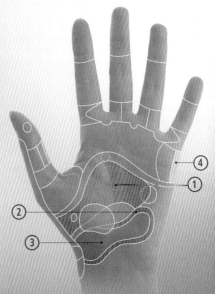

HAND ORIENTATION

LEFT HAND

Working the reflex areas in the center and heel of the palm targets organs of the digestive system as well as the upper back and arm.

The STOMACH (1) reflex area covers a large area in the center of the palm, while the COLON (2) reflex area runs across the heel of the hand, around the reflex area for the SMALL INTESTINE (3). The ARM (4) reflex area is located in the fleshy pad just below the little finger.

In general, the reflex areas on the left and right hands mirror one another exactly. However, the gall bladder and the liver reflex areas feature only on the right hand, while the stomach features only on the left.

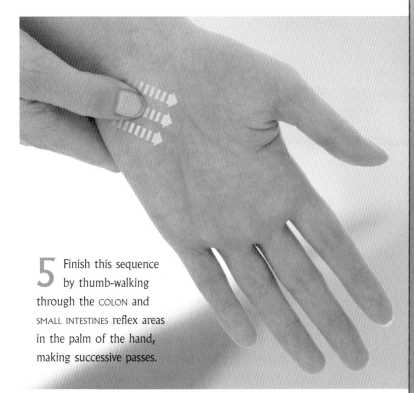

5 Finish this sequence by thumb-walking through the COLON and SMALL INTESTINES reflex areas in the palm of the hand, making successive passes.

DESSERTS   Relax your entire hand by applying the finger-pull technique to the thumb and each finger (p. 82).

STEP 5

Working the tops of the fingers and the side of the thumb

In this sequence, you work the reflex area corresponding to the spine, which includes the related nerves and muscles. Also worked are reflex areas corresponding to the head and neck, including those for the sinuses, teeth, gums, and jaw. In addition, work in this sequence relaxes the hand itself. If you encounter sensitivity in any area, thumb-walk in place or apply technique to a joint.

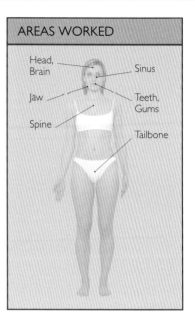

AREAS WORKED

Head, Brain
Sinus
Jaw
Teeth, Gums
Spine
Tailbone

1 To work the SPINE reflex area, thumb-walk up the bony edge of the hand, starting at the TAILBONE reflex area at the base of the thumb, near the wrist.

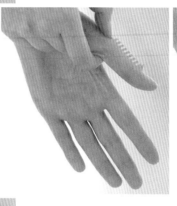

2 Continue working the SPINE reflex area, reposition your right hand and continue to thumb-walk through the midback (between the shoulder blades) reflex area. Make several passes over the joint at the base of the thumb.

3 Change your hand position and use your right thumb to thumb-walk through the NECK reflex area on the thumb, in the direction of the arrow.

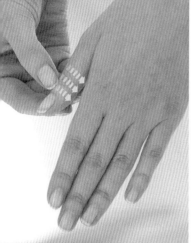

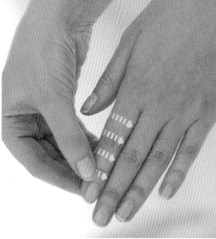

HAND ORIENTATION

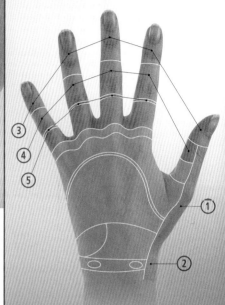

4 To work the HEAD, BRAIN, SINUS, NECK, TEETH, GUM, and JAW reflex areas, thumb-walk with your right hand across the top of the thumb several times.

5 Move on to the index finger to work the next portion of these reflex areas. Thumb-walk across the top of the finger, making a series of passes round the finger.

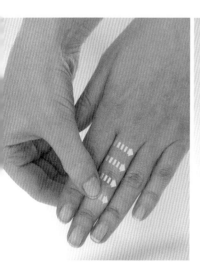

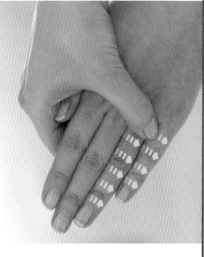

6 Continue thumb-walking, in a series of passes around the middle finger.

7 Complete this sequence by working around first the ring and then the little finger.

DESSERT   Improve circulation to the tips of your fingers with the nail-buffing technique, moving the fingernails of one hand briskly over the nails of the other hand. (p. 84)

LEFT HAND

Working the reflex areas on the tops of the fingers and the side of the thumb targets the spine and various structures of the face and head.

The reflex area for the SPINE ① runs down the outside of the thumb, with the TAILBONE ② area near the wrist. The reflex area representing the HEAD, BRAIN, and SINUS ③ occupies the first segment of each finger and thumb. Under these, on the next section of each finger and thumb, is the reflex area for the NECK ④. The reflex area for the TEETH, GUMS, and JAW ⑤ is a narrow band at the second joint on each finger.

The reflex areas on the right and left hands mirror each other exactly, those on the left hand relating to the left side of the body and those on the right hand to the right side.

STEP 6

Working the top of the hand

This sequence works the bony top of the hand, which corresponds to the musculoskeletal structure of the upper and lower body, as well as to organs of reproduction, respiration, and fluid elimination. When you have completed this sequence, which prompts an overall relaxation effect, you will have worked your way through all the reflex areas of one hand. Finish with a series of desserts.

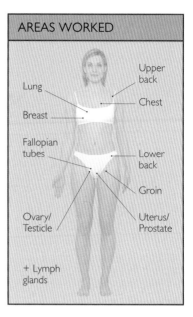

AREAS WORKED

Lung
Upper back
Chest
Breast
Fallopian tubes
Lower back
Groin
Ovary/Testicle
Uterus/Prostate

+ Lymph glands

1 Rest the flats of your fingers alongside the long bone below the index finger. Press your fingertips several times into this part of the LUNG, CHEST, BREAST, and UPPER BACK reflex areas. Move on, resting your fingertips between the index and middle finger and repeat the technique, pressing several times.

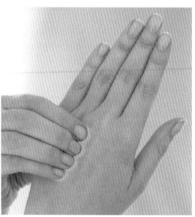

2 Reposition your fingers between the middle and ring fingers and press as before. Repeat the technique between the ring and little fingers.

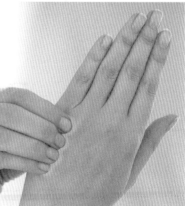

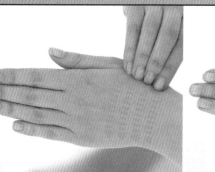

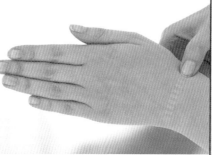

3 Now use all four fingers to finger-walk across the LOWER BACK reflex area. Repeat several times.

4 Position your right thumb on the wrist and thumb-walk through the LYMPH GLAND, GROIN, and FALLOPIAN TUBE reflex areas across the wrist.

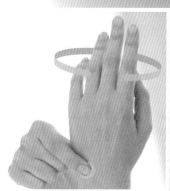

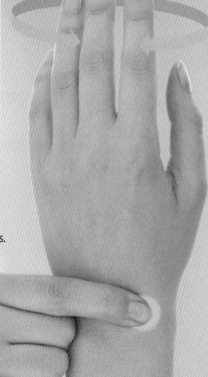

5 Pinpoint the OVARY/TESTICLE reflex area with the index finger. Rotate the hand clockwise, then counter-clockwise several times.

6 Locate the UTERUS/ PROSTATE reflex area and rotate the hand repeatedly in a clockwise then in a counter-clockwise direction.

DESSERTS   End your session by reapplying a series of desserts (p. 82–85)

HAND ORIENTATION

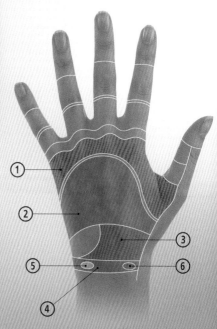

LEFT HAND

Working the top of the hand targets reflex areas relating to the musculoskeletal system, and organs of reproduction and respiration.

Close to the fingers is the reflex area for the UPPER BACK, LUNG, CHEST, and BREAST ①. Next to this is another reflex area for the UPPER BACK ②, then, nearer the wrist, the LOWER BACK ③ reflex area. In a narrow band near the wrist is the reflex area for the LYMPH GLANDS, FALLOPIAN TUBES, and GROIN ④. Within this are the reflex areas for the TESTICLE in men or the OVARY in women ⑤ and also the reflex area for the PROSTATE GLAND in men and the UTERUS in women ⑥.

The reflex areas on both hands mirror each other, with those on the left hand corresponding to the left side of the body and those on the right hand reflecting the right side.

STEP 7
Working the right hand

Now that you've given the left hand a workout, it's time to move onto the right hand. These pages show the sequence for a right hand workout. They also provide a workout summary. Once you have become familiar with how techniques are applied to each part of the hand, this summary provides an at-a-glance reminder of reflexology technique application.

DESSERTS

Before beginning the sequence, check the hand for cuts, bruises, and any other areas to be avoided during the workout

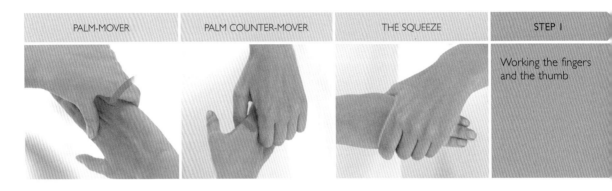

PALM-MOVER	PALM COUNTER-MOVER	THE SQUEEZE	STEP I

STEP I — Working the fingers and the thumb

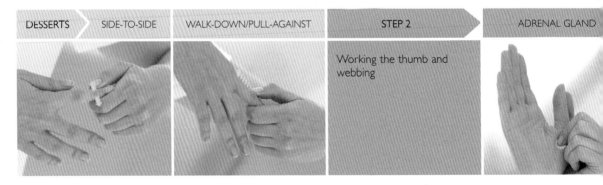

| DESSERTS > SIDE-TO-SIDE | WALK-DOWN/PULL-AGAINST | STEP 2 > | ADRENAL GLAND |

STEP 2 — Working the thumb and webbing

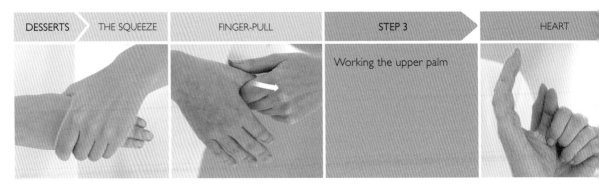

| DESSERTS > THE SQUEEZE | FINGER-PULL | STEP 3 > | HEART |

STEP 3 — Working the upper palm

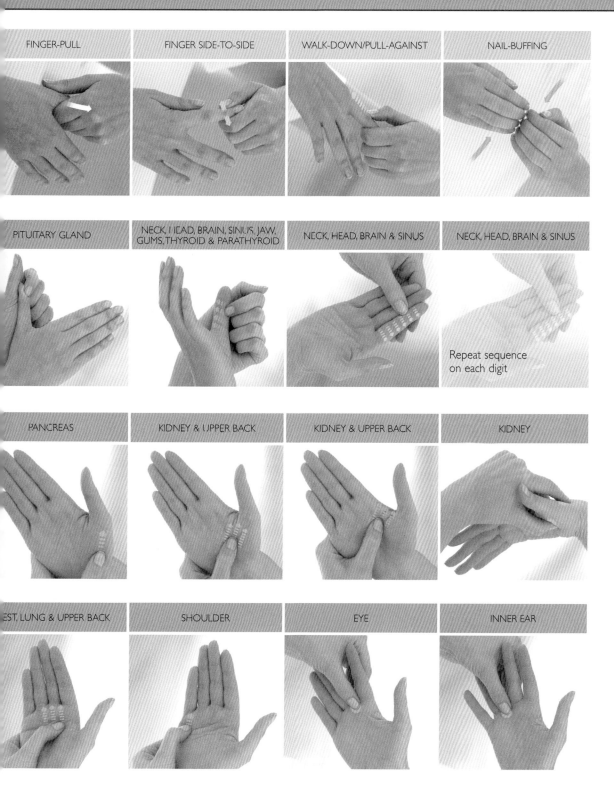

FINGER-PULL

FINGER SIDE-TO-SIDE

WALK-DOWN/PULL-AGAINST

NAIL-BUFFING

PITUITARY GLAND

NECK, HEAD, BRAIN, SINUS, JAW, GUMS, THYROID & PARATHYROID

NECK, HEAD, BRAIN & SINUS

NECK, HEAD, BRAIN & SINUS

Repeat sequence on each digit

PANCREAS

KIDNEY & UPPER BACK

KIDNEY & UPPER BACK

KIDNEY

EST, LUNG & UPPER BACK

SHOULDER

EYE

INNER EAR

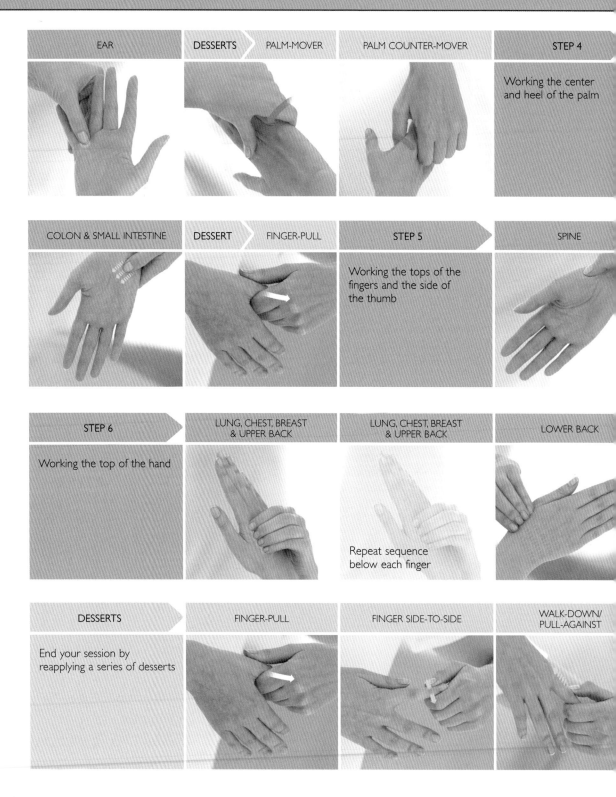

EAR

DESSERTS ❯ PALM-MOVER

PALM COUNTER-MOVER

STEP 4

Working the center and heel of the palm

COLON & SMALL INTESTINE

DESSERT ❯ FINGER-PULL

STEP 5

Working the tops of the fingers and the side of the thumb

SPINE

STEP 6

Working the top of the hand

LUNG, CHEST, BREAST & UPPER BACK

LUNG, CHEST, BREAST & UPPER BACK

Repeat sequence below each finger

LOWER BACK

DESSERTS

End your session by reapplying a series of desserts

FINGER-PULL

FINGER SIDE-TO-SIDE

WALK-DOWN/ PULL-AGAINST

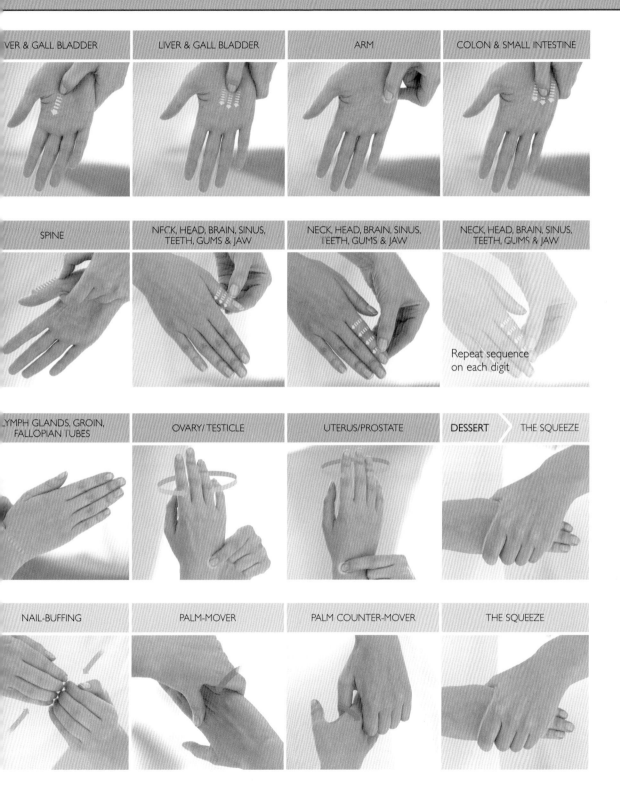

VER & GALL BLADDER

LIVER & GALL BLADDER

ARM

COLON & SMALL INTESTINE

SPINE

NECK, HEAD, BRAIN, SINUS, TEETH, GUMS & JAW

NECK, HEAD, BRAIN, SINUS, TEETH, GUMS & JAW

NECK, HEAD, BRAIN, SINUS, TEETH, GUMS & JAW

Repeat sequence on each digit

LYMPH GLANDS, GROIN, FALLOPIAN TUBES

OVARY/ TESTICLE

UTERUS/PROSTATE

DESSERT   THE SQUEEZE

NAIL-BUFFING

PALM-MOVER

PALM COUNTER-MOVER

THE SQUEEZE

STEP 1

Working the fingers and the thumb

The reflex areas worked in this sequence correspond to the head, neck, and part of the upper body. The thumb reflects the head, brain, and sinuses (first segment), neck, thyroid, and parathyroid (second segment), solar plexus, and heart reflex areas (the base). The fingers reflect the head, brain, and sinuses; neck; eyes, ears, and inner ear.

LEARNING TIP

It takes time to get accustomed to working with a golf ball so don't be too concerned about targeting the reflex area exactly as you learn. Beware of the impact of the golf ball on your hand; you will know you've overdone it if your hand becomes sensitive to the touch.

1 Starting at the base of the thumb, roll the golf ball repeatedly through the HEART reflex area. Reposition the ball and roll it over the thumb, working the NECK, THYROID, PARATHYROID, HEAD, BRAIN, and SINUS reflex areas in successive passes.

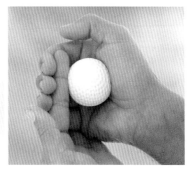

2 Go on to the index finger to continue working these reflex areas. Cup the golf ball in your hand and roll it over the index finger in successive passes until the length of the finger has been covered.

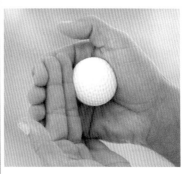

3 Go on to each finger, in turn, repeating the technique as before.

STEP 2

Working the thumb

In this sequence, you'll be working areas that correspond to organs responsible for energy and digestion – the adrenal glands, pancreas, and a portion of the stomach, liver, and intestines. This technique is uniquely capable of reaching the deep reflex areas of the palm and stimulating the functioning of vital organs. Be aware of the potential for overwork, however.

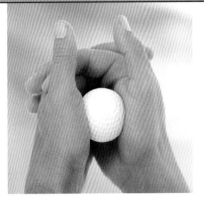

1 Interlace the fingers of the hands. and place the golf ball so that it is held securely between the heels of the hands, as shown.

2 As you roll the golf ball throughout this area of the palm, below the thumb, you are working the ADRENAL GLAND, STOMACH, PANCREAS, and KIDNEY reflex areas of both hands.

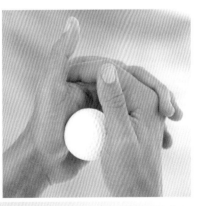

3 As you roll the golf ball, vary the pressure on the reflex areas by tightening or loosening your grasp on the ball.

STEP 3

Working the upper palm

Reflex areas worked in this sequence correspond to the upper back, shoulders, lungs, chest, and breast. Working the upper palm helps to relax the upper musculoskeletal structure, easing pain as well as stimulating and enhancing functions of the upper body.

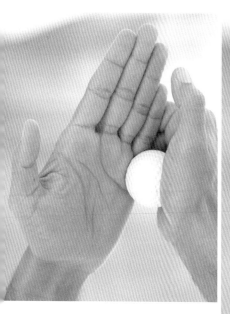

1 Reposition the golf ball so it rests in your upper palm, below the little finger. Roll the ball around the area several times, working the SHOULDER reflex area. Reposition the ball below the ring finger and roll the ball through this portion of the upper palm, working the HEART, UPPER BACK, CHEST, LUNG, and BREAST reflex areas.

2 Continue working each portion of the upper palm, successively working through the HEART, UPPER BACK, CHEST, LUNG, and BREAST reflex areas.

STEP 4

Working the center and heel of the palm

This sequence works reflex areas corresponding to organs of the body's digestive system — the stomach and spleen (left hand), liver and gall bladder (right hand), colon, and small intestines — stimulating and enhancing the functioning of those organs. Reflex areas corresponding to the back and hips are also worked, helping to create relaxation and body awareness.

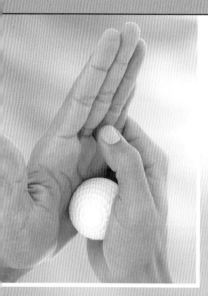

1 Position the golf ball in the center of the palm and roll it throughout the area, working the reflex areas of the UPPER BACK, STOMACH, SPLEEN, LIVER, and GALL BLADDER.

2 Next, press the golf ball between the heels of the hands and roll it throughout the reflex areas for the COLON, SMALL INTESTINE, and LOWER BACK.

STEP 5

Working the side of the thumb

This sequence works reflex areas associated with the spine, including the bony structure, the surrounding muscles, the spinal cord (which is encased by the vertebrae), and the nerves emanating from it. Work in the sequence enhances the regulatory functioning of the brain stem and spinal nerves, as well as helping to relax muscular tension in the spine.

3 Reposition the hand and golf ball, and make several passes through each part of the thumb down to the TAILBONE reflex area near the wrist.

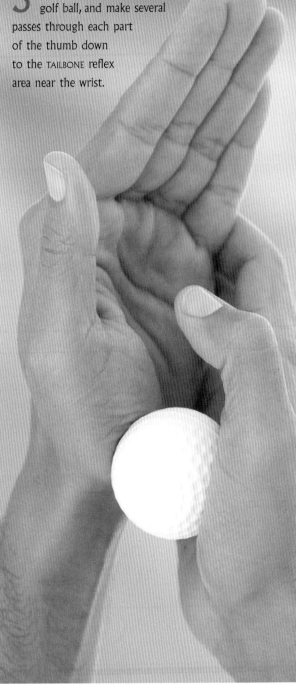

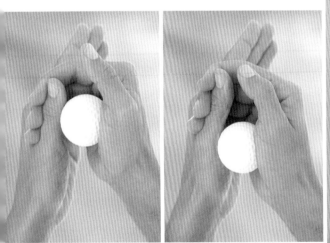

1 Position the golf ball at the NECK reflex area on the thumb, as shown. Roll the ball around, making several passes through the neck reflex area.

2 Move on to work the entire length of the bony edge of the thumb, covering the SPINE reflex area.

STEP 6

Working the fingernails

You may find that your fingernails are particularly sensitive to pressure, so work lightly to begin with. To fully work the area, roll the ball over the entire nail. Experiment with working below the nail, too, but be aware of potential sensitivity. Reflex areas in the sequence include those corresponding to the head, face, sinuses, and brain; the work will enhance brain functioning and provide relaxation.

LEARNING TIP

Note how the golf ball is held in the photos. When the thumbnail is being worked, the ball rests between the palm of the hand (below the thumb) and the nail; the thumb is braced against the fingers. When fingernails are being worked, the ball is held by the index and middle fingers of the working hand and the working thumb serves as a brace for the finger being worked.

1 Position the golf ball on the thumbnail and roll it throughout the HEAD, BRAIN, and SINUS reflex area, making several passes.

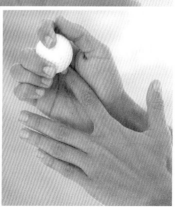

2 Continue working on each fingernail in turn, making successive passes throughout the reflex areas.

STEP 7
Working the right hand

As you've worked through the golf-ball sequence on the left hand, you've also worked many areas on the right hand, such as those in the palm. Now it's time to go on to the full sequence for the right hand, with the left hand as working hand. These pages provide both a useful workout summary and useful reminder of the complete sequence.

DESSERTS

Before beginning the sequence, check the hand for cuts, bruises, and any other areas to be avoided during the workout

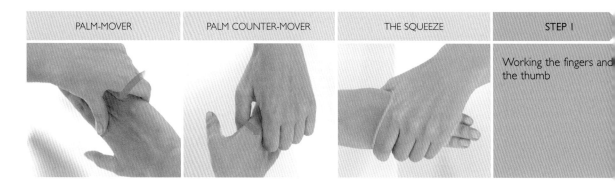

PALM-MOVER | PALM COUNTER-MOVER | THE SQUEEZE | STEP I — Working the fingers and the thumb

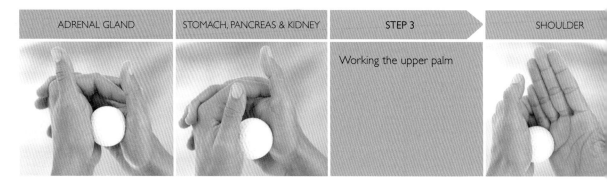

ADRENAL GLAND | STOMACH, PANCREAS & KIDNEY | STEP 3 — Working the upper palm | SHOULDER

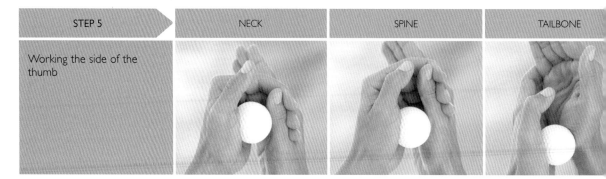

STEP 5 — Working the side of the thumb | NECK | SPINE | TAILBONE

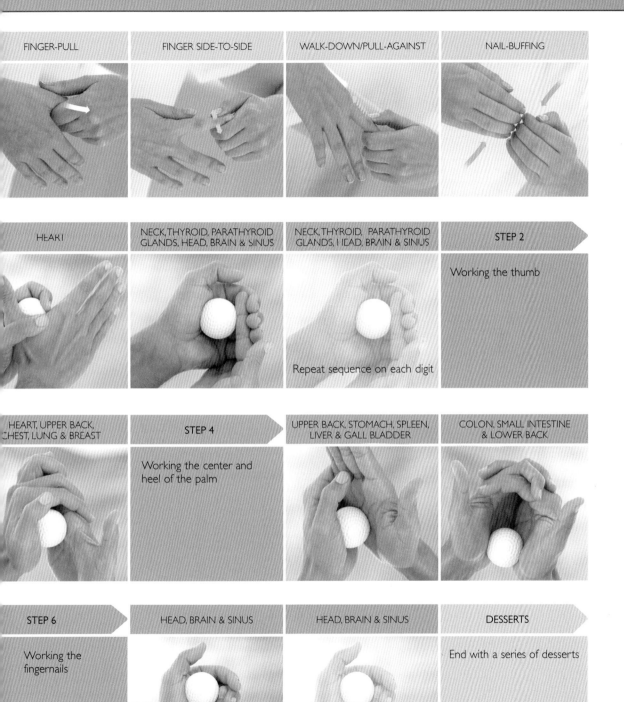

FINGER-PULL	FINGER SIDE-TO-SIDE	WALK-DOWN/PULL-AGAINST	NAIL-BUFFING

HEART	NECK, THYROID, PARATHYROID GLANDS, HEAD, BRAIN & SINUS	NECK, THYROID, PARATHYROID GLANDS, HEAD, BRAIN & SINUS	STEP 2
		Repeat sequence on each digit	Working the thumb

HEART, UPPER BACK, CHEST, LUNG & BREAST	STEP 4	UPPER BACK, STOMACH, SPLEEN, LIVER & GALL BLADDER	COLON, SMALL INTESTINE & LOWER BACK
	Working the center and heel of the palm		

STEP 6	HEAD, BRAIN & SINUS	HEAD, BRAIN & SINUS	DESSERTS
Working the fingernails		Repeat sequence on each digit	End with a series of desserts

PEOPLE WITH SPECIFIC NEEDS

Certain groups, such as babies, children, pregnant women, and the elderly, require extra consideration in reflexology work and sequences may need to be adapted for them. In general, start gently and, over the course of several sessions, gradually increase the duration of the workout and the strength of your pressure. End each session by working the kidney reflex areas to encourage the elimination of toxins.

Babies

A little reflexology goes a long way with babies and a gentle touch is needed to work tiny feet and hands. Common concerns are sleep, colic, earache, and diarrhea.

1 To calm a baby or to ease colic, press your thumb several times on the SOLAR PLEXUS / ESOPHAGUS reflex area. Repeat on both hands.

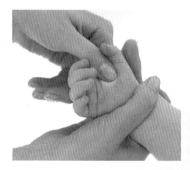

2 To ease earache, lightly pinch the EAR reflex area between your thumb and index finger.

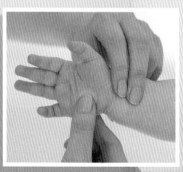

3 Gently press your thumb on the COLON reflex area to treat diarrhea. Repeat on both hands.

POINTS TO REMEMBER

Be gentle.

Work briefly with just one or two reflex areas.

To work further, gently press other reflex areas on the hand.

Children

Reflexology work with children provides a quiet time together, establishing a bond between you and encouraging relaxation. The workout outlined here targets areas of particular concern with children. Work through the reflex areas indicated, first on the right hand and then on the left, always keeping your touch light.

POINTS TO REMEMBER

Attention spans are short in young children, so don't expect to apply a full workout at this age.

Make a game of the session: for example, play *"This little piggy went to market"* while working the fingers.

A child who withdraws a hand from you is telling you something, so check carefully the reflex area and corresponding body part.

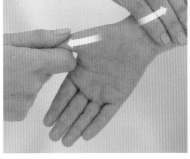

1 Lightly holding the wrist, pull gently on the thumb. Repeat on each finger and thumb in turn.

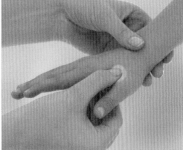

2 Holding the hand steady, gently press the SOLAR PLEXUS reflex area with the thumb of your working hand.

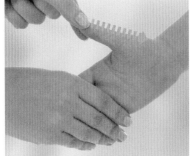

3 Thumb-walk up the SPINE reflex area of the thumb to counter the impact of the frequent falls that children inevitably experience.

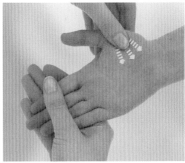

4 Reposition the thumb and thumb-walk repeatedly through the PANCREAS reflex area to help regulate the function of this organ.

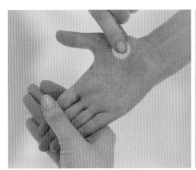

5 Pinpoint the ADRENAL GLAND reflex area and press gently with your index finger, to help regulate hormone levels.

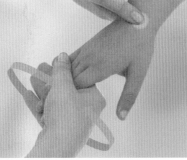

6 Pressing gently on the UTERUS/ PROSTATE reflex area, turn the hand first in a clockwise then in a counter-clockwise direction.

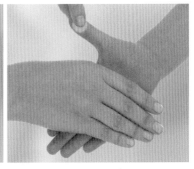

7 Finish by pressing gently and repeatedly on the PITUITARY GLAND reflex area to stimulate the body's "master gland."

Pregnant women

The concerns of pregnant women vary throughout the pregnancy, so establish an appropriate goal for each workout. For example, your session may address the need for general relaxation or to soothe an aching lower back.

To promote general relaxation

1 Enclose the thumb within the working hand and pull gently, holding for several seconds. Turn the thumb in a clockwise and then in a counter-clockwise direction. Repeat on each finger in turn.

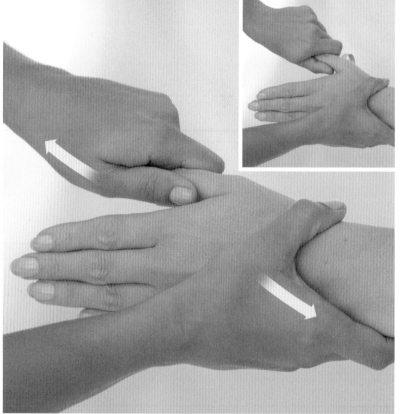
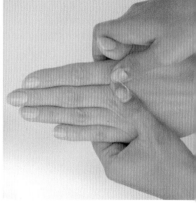

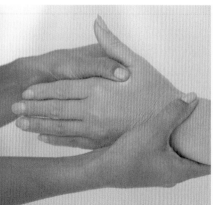
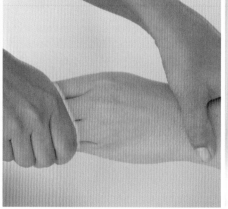
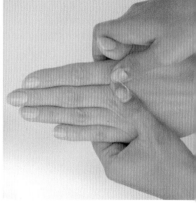

2 Locate the SOLAR PLEXUS reflex area in the webbing between thumb and index finger and press gently. Continue by pressing gently in all parts of the webbing of each hand.

3 With your working hand contoured around the recipient's hand, gently squeeze the hand several times. Move your hand along the length of the hand as you continue squeezing.

4 Rest your thumbs on top of the hand, and start moving the long bones with one thumb and counter-moving with the other. Repeat several times, to encourage gentle relaxation.

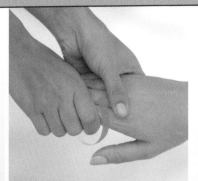

To soothe an aching lower back

1 Hold the hand as shown and press gently on the long bone below the middle finger. Repeat on each long bone, then apply the palm counter-mover technique.

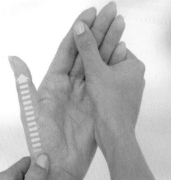

2 To work the LOWER BACK reflex area, thumb-walk through the bony heel of the hand.

3 Holding the hand steady, make a series of multiple finger-walking passes over the hand to target the LOWER BACK reflex.

4 Locate the ADRENAL REFLEX area on the heel of the hand and press gently. Repeat several times to improve general muscle tone and relieve tension.

Self-help workout

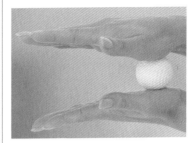

To give your hand a general workout, start by rolling a golf ball throughout the heel of the hand. Targeted reflex areas include ADRENAL GLANDS (for energy), PANCREAS (for fatigue), and STOMACH. Go on to roll the golf ball throughout the COLON reflex area. For general relaxation, finish by working the SOLAR PLEXUS reflex area in the webbing between your thumb and index finger.

CAUTION

Whether or not it is safe to apply reflexology work to pregnant women in the first trimester is a matter of debate within the profession. Our view is that reflexology is beneficial if you:

Start gradually, working for a short time and with a light touch.

Avoid repeated or extended work to any one reflex area.

Work on the kidney reflex area to encourage the elimination of toxins.

Encourage consultation with a doctor if any irregularities appear.

REFLEXOLOGY AT THE OFFICE

When you're feeling under par, the work day can seem endless. However your reflexology skills can help improve both your sense of well-being and your ability to cope with work. The reflex areas worked in this sequence are aimed at boosting your energy levels and helping you cope with stress, while other techniques are designed to relieve hands that are tired from the work they've done.

SIDESTEPPING STRESS

Stress contributes to many physical disorders, including repetitive stress injuries of the hands. It is a good idea to run through a sequence of reflexology techniques that meet your needs at regular intervals throughout the day. This will help break up habitual stress patterns and ease tension when you feel stressed. Keep a golf ball in your desk drawer and run through some techniques for a quick pick-me-up. (see *pages 102–109*).

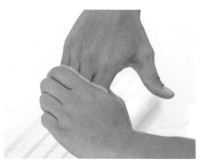

1 Clasp the hand and squeeze firmly several times. Repeat along the length of the hand.

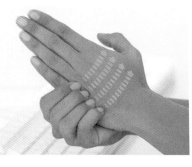

2 Apply multiple finger-walking across the back of the hand. Repeat on the opposite hand.

3 Interlace your fingers with a golf ball between your palms. Roll the ball repeatedly through the PANCREAS reflex area to help keep energy levels constant.

4 Relieve office-related tension and revive overworked hands with the application of the finger-pull dessert (*see page 82*). Repeat on each finger and thumb, on both hands.

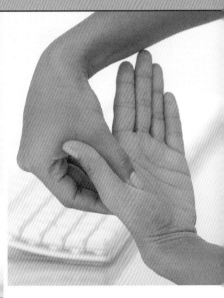

5 To promote relaxation, gently press the SOLAR PLEXUS reflex area. Reposition your thumb and finger and then press another area of the webbing.

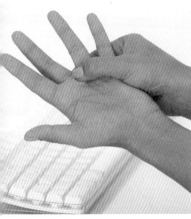

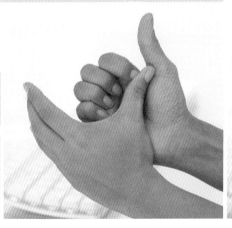

6 To relieve tension in the tops of the shoulders, a common area for stress, pinch the TOPS OF SHOULDERS reflex area in the webbing several times.

7 Targeting the HEAD reflex area can both relieve a headache and help mental alertness. Rest your fingertip in the center of the thumb and press. Repeat on each finger in turn.

8 Finally, to relax the neck, apply the side-to-side technique to the thumb. Repeat on each finger and thumb then again on the other hand.

REFLEXOLOGY ON THE MOVE

Why not use commuting time to improve your well-being? By discreetly applying a few hand-reflexology techniques during your journey, you can prepare yourself for the busy day ahead or wind down for the evening. Even if you travel by car, opportunities may arise — for example, stalled traffic or waiting at red lights — for a quick reflexology workout. Try the following exercises, which target common commuter concerns and some specific health concerns.

USING COMMUTING TIME

What health improvement would you like to see? Decide what you need to work on and use your daily commuting time to move toward achieving your goal. The great advantage of hand reflexology is that reflex areas can be worked on discreetly at any time and any place. Problems such as chronic neckache, sore hands, digestive problems, or generalized anxiety can all be targeted during your journey each morning and evening.

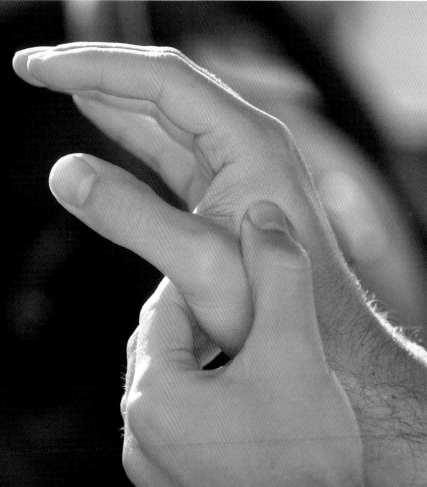

1 To help you relax, rest your thumb and fingertip in the SOLAR PLEXUS reflex area of the webbing. Pinch the thumb and fingertip together several times. Repeat on the other hand.

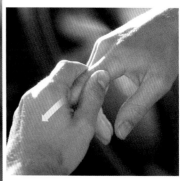

2 Apply the finger-pull dessert to both relax the fingers and work the NECK reflex area. Repeat on each finger. Change hands and repeat the sequence on the other hand.

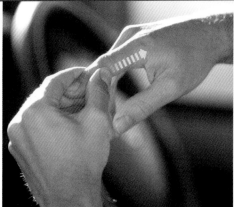

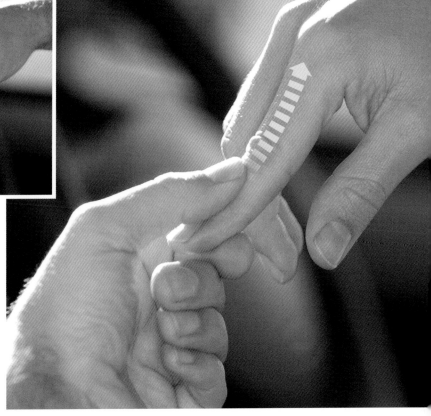

3 Apply the walk-down/pull-against technique to each finger in turn. This technique gently stretches fingers that are tired from keyboard overuse, as well as relaxing the NECK reflex area.

4 Now thumb-walk down the top of the finger, pulling it upward as you work. Repeat on each finger and the other hand.

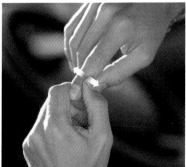

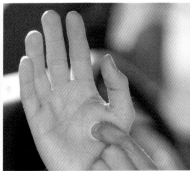

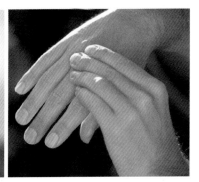

5 The finger side-to-side technique promotes flexibility in the fingers and gives them a break from the usual patterns of movement. Repeat on each finger and thumb on both hands.

6 Apply pressure to the ADRENAL GLAND reflex area to help you relax. Rock your working hand from side to side as you press with the index finger. Repeat on the other hand.

7 Keep your lower back happy by applying the palm-mover technique, first to one hand and then to the other. Counter the stretch with the palm counter-mover.

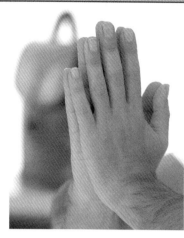

REFLEXOLOGY ON THE ROAD

Whenever you travel for business or for pleasure, it's useful to have a few reflexology techniques ready for any health concerns that may crop up. Digestive upsets, energy lags, insomnia, and musculoskeletal aches are all common occurrences when traveling. Keep in mind those hand reflexology dessert techniques to ease joints and muscles aching from hours of cramped air travel or an unfamiliar bed.

1 Place your palms together and press for several seconds; then link your fingers and push outward, holding for several seconds.

2 Place one hand on top of the other, as shown, and press down. Reverse hands and repeat.

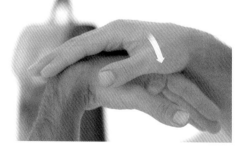

3 To address digestive concerns, roll a golf ball throughout the DIGESTIVE reflex areas in the heels of the hands. Alternatively, thumb-walk throughout the reflex areas.

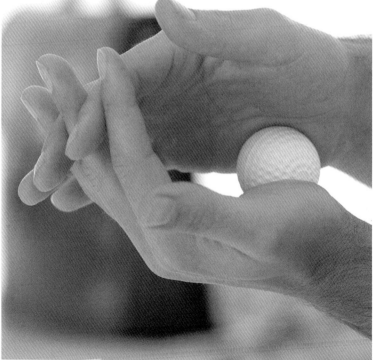

TRAVELING TIPS

Take along a golf ball for quick reflexology fixes on the road. Lightweight and portable, the golf ball is the perfect on-the-road self-help companion.

If you're trying to sleep, try the relaxing properties of hands soaked for several minutes in warm water.

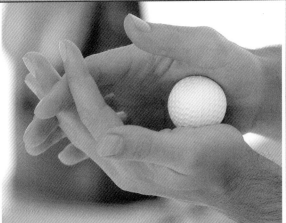

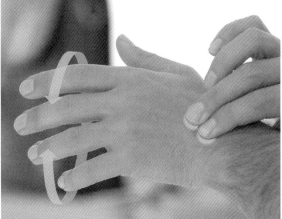

4 Revive flagging energy by rolling a golf ball through the PANCREAS and ADRENAL GLAND reflex areas in the heel of the hands. Or use the hook and back-up technique to work on the reflex areas.

5 Ease the stress of sitting for long periods by targeting LOWER BACK reflex area. Rest two fingers on top of the hand and the thumb underneath, then rotate the hand clockwise then counter-clockwise.

6 Next apply the palm-mover to relax both the upper and lower back.

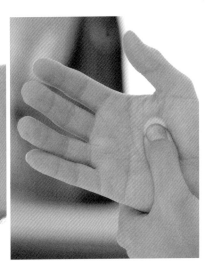

7 To help you relax before sleeping, apply pressure to the SOLAR PLEXUS reflex area. Gently pinch the webbing of the hand, paying particular attention to any part that is sensitive.

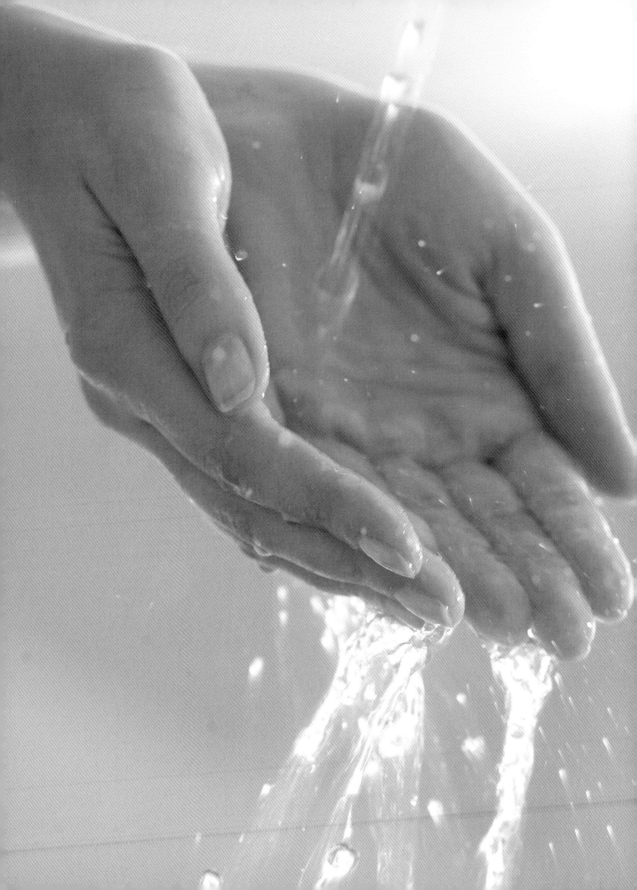

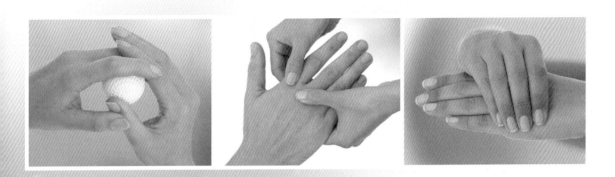

REFLEXOLOGY TO TARGET HEALTH CONCERNS

From easing backache to boosting low energy or refreshing tired hands, reflexology provides a safe and convenient adjunct to standard medical treatment. In this chapter, we present in-depth advice on addressing a number of disorders and health concerns, with descriptions of techniques and reflex areas appropriate to each.

USING REFLEXOLOGY FOR HEALTH CONCERNS

Applying reflexology work to the whole hand prompts overall relaxation and a sense of well-being as well as relaxing the hand itself. When addressing specific health concerns, technique application is focused on specific reflex areas corresponding to the parts or organs of the body that are giving rise to concern. In this case, those specific reflex areas can be worked on following a general workout or — if time is short or the problem acute — they can be targeted in a specially tailored mini-session.

When planning a mini-session to target a specific health concern, focus attention on the reflex area that corresponds to the particular area of concern. For some concerns, the selection of reflex areas will follow the reflexology chart: for example, if the health concern is with the function of the lungs — as, for instance, with disorders such as asthma, emphysema, and bronchitis — then the reflexology work will target the lung reflex.

In addition to the primary reflex area, however, additional reflexes may be chosen for their impact on the particular health concerns. For example, as well as working the lung reflex area, the adrenal reflex gland may also be targeted to help relieve the symptoms of bronchitis. The adrenal glands are responsible for producing hormones that are needed for fighting inflammation, so work applied to this reflex area may prompt speedier healing.

WORKING ROUND THE CONCERN

Stress is a factor in some 80 percent of health concerns and, in those cases, reflex areas corresponding to the body's tension spots are targeted for additional technique emphasis. When planning a mini-session to relieve an upset digestive system, for example, the solar plexus reflex area (which can be worked to relieve tension and stress) will be included along with the reflex areas of the stomach, small intestine, and colon.

As you apply reflexology techniques, take note of which reflex areas give the best results. You may find a particular combination of reflex areas that works best for you. If you find that work on a specific part of the hand feels good, apply extra technique there. Particularly with self-help reflexology work, experiment with reflex areas, techniques, and random parts of the hand — or with areas to which you find yourself drawn.

REFLEXOLOGY STRATEGIES

There are no hard and fast rules for deciding how much and how often to apply technique. A series of strategies, however, will help you get the best results. Think in terms of working and applying technique to relevant reflex areas until the problem subsides. For example, to deal with a cold, work the adrenal gland reflex areas when the sniffles appear and continue until they abate.

Alternatively you might prefer to set a time and place, such as working for five minutes at breakfast, lunch, and dinner. This will give your work the consistency that is key in getting results.

Another successful strategy is to get into the habit of applying reflexology technique whenever you have a few spare minutes. Talking on the telephone, stopping at a traffic light, or waiting for an appointment all offer opportunities that can be usefully employed: you will find that accumulated small chunks of time add up.

CAUTIONS

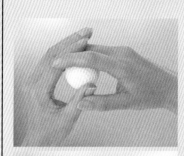

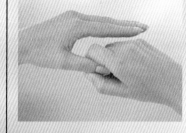

If you have a health problem, consult a physician before starting work: reflexology is an adjunct to medical care, not a substitute.

If you are pregnant, be aware of the specific cautions that apply (see *pages 112–113*).

When working with babies, children, or the elderly, work more frequently but with less pressure and for a shorter period of time.

When working the pancreas reflex area of individuals with diabetes or hypoglycemia, work only lightly and briefly to begin.

When working with someone who is severely ill, work only for brief periods of time, applying light pressure and be sure to stay within the recipient's comfort zone.

If a part of the hand feels sensitive to the touch after reflexology work, it may have been overworked. Let the area rest for a few days and when you begin work again, work for a shorter amount of time and with less pressure.

Do not overwork a reflex area that reflects an infected body part; for example, the lung reflex area of the hand in someone with bronchitis.

ADDRESSING HEALTH CONCERNS

DEAL WITH STRESS: Studies show that stress and tension contribute to the majority of health concerns. Make a point, therefore, of addressing such concerns with one of the following three strategies:
1. Give the hand a complete workout or, better still, have someone else do it: a workout from someone else is more relaxing than working on oneself.
2. Indulge your hands in a session of nothing but desserts (*see pages 60–65 and 82–85*).
3. Apply technique repeatedly to the solar plexus reflex area, especially at the beginning and end of a session.

"FEEL-GOOD" FACTOR: People often say "That feels good" during a workout. Take note of the area or dessert and remember to work with it more often in the future.

WORK WITHIN THE COMFORT ZONE: Remember that the primary aim of a workout is relaxation, so make sure you stay within a recipient's comfort zone.

DRINK WATER: It is important to drink lots of water after a workout, to help rid the body of toxins. Aid this by focusing on the kidney reflex area in the first few sessions.

STRESS

In the vast majority of health concerns, stress plays a contributory role. Reflexology, however, provides a safe and effective method of general stress control, as well as a means of easing the impact of stress on specific parts of your body. For general stress reduction, work on the solar plexus and the adrenal gland reflex areas (*see pages 16–17*), applying the technique for longer periods of time until you achieve relief.

RESEARCH

Researchers in Singapore have demonstrated that reflexology impacts on areas of the brain involved in relaxation. Using electro-encephalography (EEG) to record brain activity, they showed that the application of reflexology technique to the brain reflex area of the thumb produced brain activity consistent with relaxation.

Working the hands

Target the adrenal gland and solar plexus reflex areas for a general relaxation effect. When working the solar plexus reflex, enhance the effect by pressing and holding the pressure in place for a few seconds.

1 Clasp the recipient's wrist with your right hand to keep the hand steady. Pinch the webbing between thumb and finger, pressing repeatedly on the ADRENAL GLAND reflex area with the tip of the index finger.

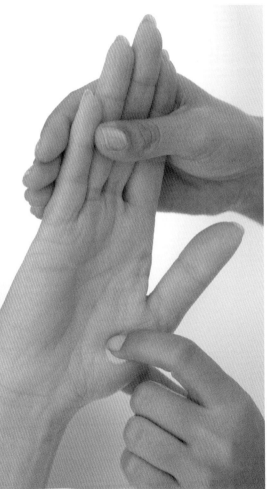

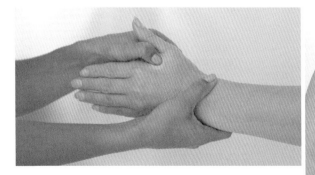

2 To find the SOLAR PLEXUS reflex area, straighten the fingers of the right hand. Place the tip of your left index finger in the center of the fleshy palm, midway along the long bone below the thumb. Press repeatedly.

Self-help hand reflexology

The solar plexus and adrenal gland reflex areas are easily accessible, making this an easy and convenient stress-relieving technique that you can use anywhere, any time. Apply the technique as often as needed to obtain relief.

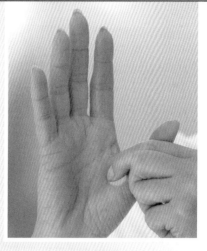

1 Locate the ADRENAL GLAND reflex area with the tip of your left index finger, midway along the long bone below the thumb. Press repeatedly with your index finger.

2 Gripping the hand between the thumb and index finger, press repeatedly on the SOLAR PLEXUS reflex area with the flat of the index finger.

OVERALL STRESS REDUCTION

One strategy for dealing with stress is to apply a general hand-relaxation technique: when your hands relax, your whole body relaxes, improving its response to stress as well as benefiting specific areas. Techniques include:

Paraffin bath (see page 53)

Using a foot-roller as a hand-roller

Hand-rolling techniques (spiky balls)

Applying golf-ball techniques

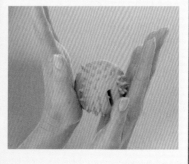

HEADACHES

Tension is often implicated in headaches, but it's worth experimenting with the sequences below to see what works best. The chart opposite recommends reflex areas and technique for different types of headache according to whether the problem is a migraine headache or pain in a particular part of the head.

RESEARCH

A Danish study in 1997 found that reflexology helped ease headaches. Most importantly, many participants came to think of "working on" their headaches rather than just "living with" them. The study concluded: "The patients see themselves as vital agents in the process of illness and of curing themselves."

Working the hands

Neck tension frequently contributes to headaches, and working the neck reflex areas may relieve this. Work both hands evenly, repeating the movements on each digit and thumb in turn. Seek out sensitive areas, as working on these can help to relieve pain and tension.

1 To relieve tension, work the NECK and HEAD reflex areas, using the walk-down/pull-against dessert (*see page 64*). The fingertips work against the thumb to create leverage and stretch the finger.

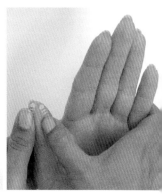

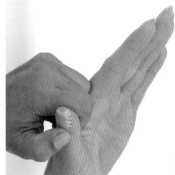

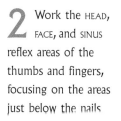

2 Work the HEAD, FACE, and SINUS reflex areas of the thumbs and fingers, focusing on the areas just below the nails

3 Now apply the thumb-walking technique to work the HEAD and BRAIN reflex areas on the thumb and fingers.

Self-help hand reflexology

If you develop a headache, identify what type it is and where the pain is located. Check the chart below, which lists different types of headache, then apply the appropriate technique to the suggested reflex area.

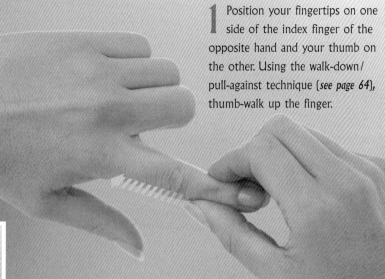

1 Position your fingertips on one side of the index finger of the opposite hand and your thumb on the other. Using the walk-down/pull-against technique (*see page 64*), thumb-walk up the finger.

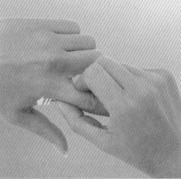

2 Reposition your hand and target the joint, thumb-walking down the side of the finger while stretching the inside edge. Repeat this sequence on each of the fingers in turn.

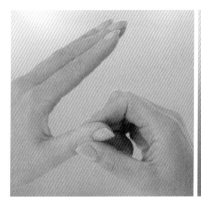

3 Holding your thumb as shown between thumb and index finger, exert pressure for several seconds. Repeat across the thumb, repositioning the working thumb and pressing the area below the nail.

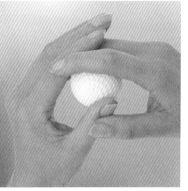

4 Rest the thumb on the golf ball as shown. Roll the golf ball over the HEAD reflex area by rocking the hand back and forth. Repeat on the first segment of each finger of both hands.

TYPES OF HEADACHE

Depending on the nature of your headache and location of the pain, work the following reflex areas with the suggested techniques:

MIGRAINE HEADACHE: Thumb-walk along the SPINE reflex area.

MIGRAINE HEADACHE WITH VISION IMPAIRMENT: Walk-down/pull-against through the NECK reflex area on the index finger.

HEADACHE AT TOP OF HEAD: Work the HEAD reflex area on the first segment of the digits.

HEADACHE AT SIDE OF HEAD: Work the HEAD reflex on the sides of the thumb.

PAIN AT BACK OF HEAD: Thumb-walk the HEAD reflex area on the first segment of the thumb.

BACKACHE & NECK PAIN

Working to alleviate pain starts with identifying where the pain is located in the body then using hand maps (*see pages 16–19*) to identify the corresponding reflex areas. As you apply technique to these areas, look out for particularly sensitive areas, which usually correspond closely with the location of the pain in the body.

RESEARCH

Chinese researchers demonstrated pain reduction following reflexology work in those suffering from degeneration of cervical disks. Another study found that reflexology lessened pain in a group of 40 persons suffering from herniated lumbo-sacral disks.

Working the hands

It is best to apply technique to a broad portion of the relevant reflex area. To work the spine reflex area, for example, make a series of passes to one side of the reflex area, followed by one down the center, and then one slightly to either side.

1 To relieve tension in the NECK, hold the thumb steady below the first joint with the holding hand, then apply the side-to-side technique (*see page 63*). Move the thumb several times then repeat the action on each finger.

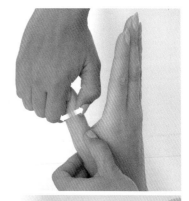

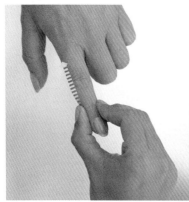

2 Thumb-walk down the side of the index finger through the NECK reflex area. Make several passes over each joint then reposition and repeat on each finger in turn.

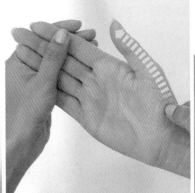

3 Hold the hand in place and thumb-walk up the SPINE reflex area, making several passes over a broad area of the thumb. Reposition the walking thumb as necessary.

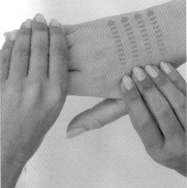

4 Hold the fingers to steady the hand and apply the multiple finger-walking technique to the back of the hand. Cover the entire area with successive passes.

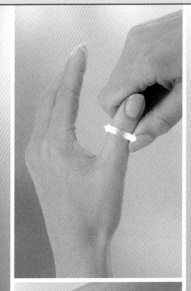

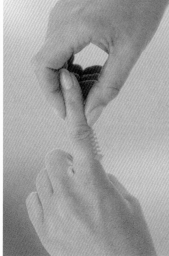

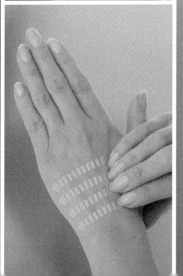

Self-help hand reflexology

From the sequences below, choose the one that seems most appropriate to your particular back or neck pain. In time you will become more aware of which technique or particular reflex area works for you and you can then work discreetly on the area as frequently as you require.

1 To work the NECK reflex area, apply the side-to-side technique to the thumb joints, moving each joint several times. Repeat on the joints of the other fingers.

2 Continue work on the NECK reflex area. On the index finger, apply the walk-down/pull-against technique, making several passes, especially over the second joint. Repeat on the third joint (the knuckle of the hand). Repeat the work on each finger.

3 To target LOWER BACK, HIP, or KNEE concerns, apply multiple finger-walking to the back of the hand, making several passes. Reposition the working hand closer to the wrist and repeat.

4 Begin by thumb-walking up the SPINE reflex area of the hand, making multiple passes. Then target the portion corresponding to your concern and apply more technique.

PAIN

In hand reflexology, pain is addressed by identifying the relevant reflex area, then applying a direct, steady, constant pressure until the pain eases. Working the solar plexus reflex and applying hand desserts also help to ease the general tension levels. However, you should always have any unknown pain diagnosed by your doctor.

RESEARCH

Numerous studies have shown that reflexology provides pain relief for cancer patients, the elderly, and patients recovering from surgery, as well as relieving headaches and toothache. Research has also shown that reflexology relieves pain in patients with kidney stones.

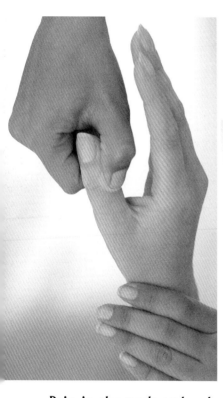

Working the hands

The following are suggestions for easing pain in the head, neck, chest, and abdomen, and for easing tension. Experiment to see which part of the reflex area being worked relates most closely to the pain.

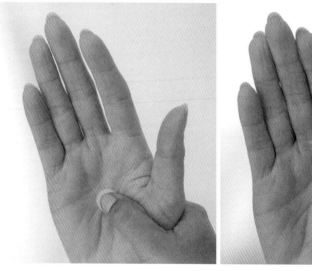

Pain in the neck or head

Apply direct pressure to the HEAD and NECK reflex area in the thumb or finger by squeezing the digit as shown. Hold for 15–30 seconds. Experiment by working different portions of different fingers, to find what works best.

Pain in abdomen or chest

If the pain is in the trunk of the body, work the palm of the hand. For chest pain, work the upper palm or base of the thumb. Press with the thumb, holding for 15–30 seconds. Reposition your thumb to search out the most sensitive area.

To relieve tension

Place your thumb and fingertip in the webbing at the SOLAR PLEXUS reflex area. Press repeatedly, holding for 15–30 seconds. Reposition and work on another segment of the webbing, to relax the upper back. Search out the most sensitive area.

Self-help hand reflexology

Because the hand is so accessible,
it is easy to apply self-help
reflexology techniques for
easing pain. In addition,
you will find out which
area is the most sensitive
and thus where to
focus your efforts.

For pain in the neck or head

Apply pressure to the HEAD or NECK
reflex area on the thumb or fingers,
holding for 15–30 seconds. Search out the
most sensitive area and focus your attention there.

WHERE DOES IT HURT?

Note the location of the pain then
find the corresponding reflex area
on the hand. Remember that the
left side of the body is reflected on
the left hand and the right side of
the body on the right hand. The
waistline is reflected at the base of
the long bones of the hands (see
page 39), while the reflex area
corresponding to the tops of the
shoulders is located at the base of
the fingers. The thumb reflects the
body's center line, while the outer
aspect of the hand reflects the
outer aspect of the body.

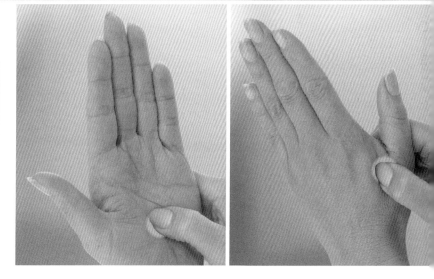

Pain in abdomen or chest

For pain in the trunk of the body,
work the palm of the hand; for
chest pain, work the upper palm
or base of the thumb. Press with the
thumb, holding for 15–30 seconds.
Experiment until you find the
most sensitive area.

To relieve tension

Place the thumb and fingertips in
the webbing of the hand as shown
above. Press together, holding for
15–30 seconds. Reposition the
thumb and finger then again press
for 15–30 seconds. Repeat the
work throughout the webbing.

BREAST CANCER RECOVERY

Coping with chemotherapy and its physical effects, as well as with the emotional toll of receiving a diagnosis of breast cancer, have all been successfully addressed through the use of reflexology. Targeted reflex areas include: the chest, lungs, and breast; the adrenal glands (addressing the fight or flight aspect of stress); the solar plexus (to encourage relaxation); and the lymphatic glands (because of the relationship with breast tissue).

RESEARCH

Many studies have documented the positive impact of reflexology on women undergoing treatment for breast cancer. Symptoms such as nausea, vomiting, anxiety, and pain have been reduced or relieved, helping women to adjust better to their diagnosis and treatment. Researchers have also found that reflexology brings about a decrease in depression and improvement in emotional quality of life in women diagnosed with breast cancer.

Working the hands

The reflex areas for the chest, lungs, and breast and the solar plexus span the broad expanse of the upper palm, including the top of the hand. The adrenal gland reflex area is a pinpoint, while the lymphatic gland reflex extends around the top of the wrist. Apply desserts frequently, as touch alone is important.

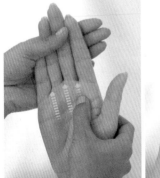

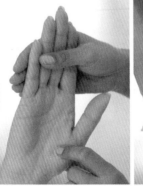

1 To work the CHEST, LUNG, BREAST, and SOLAR PLEXUS reflex areas, hold the fingers back and apply a series of passes through the upper palm.

2 Reposition the working hand to pinpoint the ADRENAL GLAND reflex area with the tip of the index finger and press repeatedly.

3 Turn the hand over and thumb-walk over the CHEST, LUNG, BREAST, and SOLAR PLEXUS reflex areas on the top of the hand.

4 Holding the recipient's hand straight with the holding hand, start finger-walking through the LYMPHATIC GLAND reflex area around the wrist.

Self-help hand reflexology

While there are benefits to receiving hand reflexology from another person, research has shown that self-applied reflexology can also result in relaxation. As well as the techniques shown below, consider using the general relaxation exercises (*see pages 46–47*) as well as self-help desserts (*see pages 82–85*).

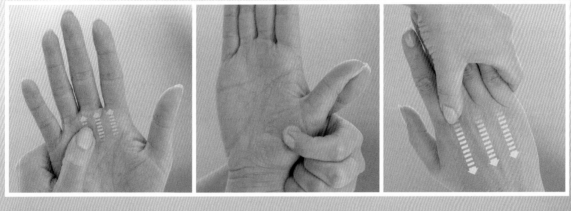

1 Hold your hand palm side up and thumb-walk in successive passes through the CHEST, LUNG, BREAST, and SOLAR PLEXUS reflex areas.

2 Locate the ADRENAL GLAND reflex area and press repeatedly.

3 Turn your hand over and thumb-walk down the CHEST, LUNG, BREAST and SOLAR PLEXUS reflex areas on the top of the hand.

4 Continue working on the back of the hand, finger-walking around the LYMPHATIC GLAND reflex area in the wrist area.

THE DESSERT SESSION

For the ultimate in relaxation, nothing beats a session of dessert techniques (*see pages 60–65* and *82–85*). Whether self-administered or applied by another, desserts relax the hands and address the recipient's overall tension pattern.

OTHER HEALTH CONCERNS

Unless otherwise stated, apply techniques 3–4 times a day, several minutes at a time, then switch hands. Every health concern listed in this section provides at least one self-help technique: these are denoted by a cross (✛) in the top right-hand corner of the picture.

Low energy & fatigue

Reduced energy levels, especially late in the day, can be the result of low blood-sugar levels. Since the pancreas is involved in regulating blood-sugar levels, working the pancreas reflex area 3–4 times a day may help the condition. Working the adrenal gland reflex areas may also help to improve the production of adrenaline and thereby increase energy levels.

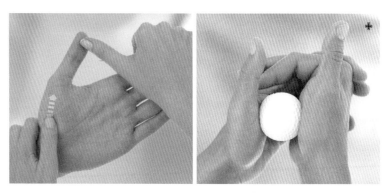

Thumb-walk through the PANCREAS reflex area, making a series of successive passes.

Roll a golf ball through the PANCREAS and ADRENAL GLAND reflex areas for 2 minutes.

Asthma

An allergic condition of the lungs, asthma is associated with breathing difficulty and wheezing. Adrenaline, produced by the adrenal glands, is thought to help the lungs relax and facilitate normal breathing. Working the adrenal gland reflex areas 3–4 times a day may help to relieve asthmatic symptoms since it improves adrenaline production.

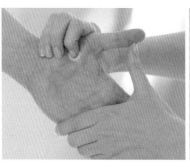

Pinpoint the ADRENAL GLAND reflex area with the index finger and press gently several times.

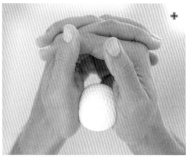

Hold a golf ball between the heels of the hands. Roll it through the ADRENAL GLAND reflex areas.

Allergies & hay fever

Hay fever is an allergic response to pollen, but other allergies can be triggered by a variety of things. A common symptom of all allergies, however, is inflammation. Cortisol, a hormone secreted by the adrenal glands, may reduce levels of the chemical that causes inflammation. To ease allergic symptoms, work the adrenal gland reflex area 3–4 times a day.

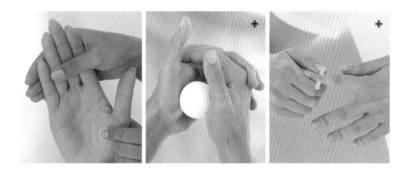

Locate the ADRENAL GLAND reflex area and press gently several times. Repeat 3–4 times daily.

Rest a golf ball between the hands, as shown, and roll it through the ADRENAL GLAND reflex areas.

Sinus problems & headaches

Sinus problems and headaches are often the result of excess mucus clogging the sinus cavities. Working the adrenal gland reflex areas may help to relieve the symptoms associated with these conditions. In addition, you can also try the side-to-side dessert, which may help to unclog the sinus cavities and ease symptoms.

Gently press the ADRENAL GLAND reflex areas several times.

Roll a golf ball through the ADRENAL GLAND reflex areas for several minutes.

Grasp the sides of each finger joint and move it gently from side to side.

High blood pressure

Stress is a major contributing factor in high blood pressure, but targeted reflexology techniques may help to reduce stress levels. To help improve the body's stress response, target the reflex areas for the adrenal gland. Working the solar plexus reflex area will help to bring about a state of calm. Apply technique 3–4 times a day.

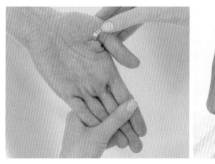

Thumb-walk through the ADRENAL GLAND reflex area, making several passes. Repeat throughout the day.

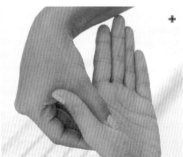

Pinch the SOLAR PLEXUS reflex area in the webbing of the thumb. Repeat several times during the day.

Anxiety & depression

At the very least, conditions such as anxiety and depression require relaxation. To induce a sense of calm, work the solar plexus reflex area. Target the pancreas reflex area to help stabilize the blood-sugar levels, and work the adrenal gland reflex areas to normalize adrenaline production.

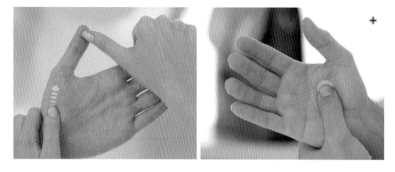

Thumb-walk through the PANCREAS and ADRENAL GLAND reflex areas. Repeat 3–4 times each day.

Gently pinch the SOLAR PLEXUS reflex area, as shown, holding for several minutes. Repeat 3–4 times per day.

Heart problems

For heart conditions, work the heart reflex area, the adrenal gland reflex area (to improve adrenaline production), and the brain reflex area (parts of the brain regulate some of the heart's activities) 3–4 times a day.

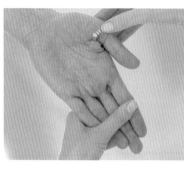
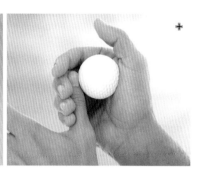

Thumb-walk around the base of the thumb, making multiple passes to cover the HEART reflex area.

Grip a golf ball in your fingers. Roll it back and forth through the BRAIN reflex area.

Incontinence

The body's inability to control urination is known as incontinence. Since parts of the brain are involved in controlling this basic bodily function, working the brain reflex area may help to improve the condition.

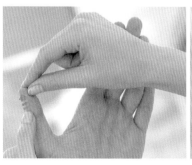
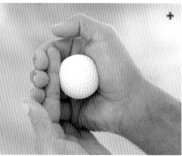

Thumb-walk several times through the BRAIN reflex area on the edge of the thumb. Repeat on each digit.

Roll a golf ball through the BRAIN reflex area on the side of the index finger. Repeat on each digit.

Fluid retention

The kidneys are responsible for regulating the body's water needs and eliminating waste products. Reduced blood flow to the kidneys can result in fluid retention. Target the kidney reflex area to help ease fluid retention.

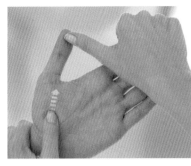

Thumb-walk through the KIDNEY reflex area, making several successive passes.

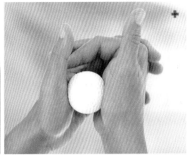

Rest a golf ball in the palm of the hand, just under the thumb, and roll through the KIDNEY reflex area.

Stroke

A stroke results from an interruption in the brain's blood supply (often as a result of a blood vessel rupture). Strokes can lead to paralysis, unconsciousness, and other problems. Apply technique for several minutes, 3–4 times a day, to the brain reflex area on the side of the body opposite the side that is paralyzed.

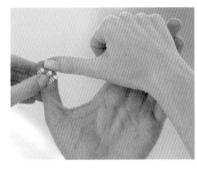

Hold the thumb steady as you thumb-walk through the BRAIN reflex area for several minutes.

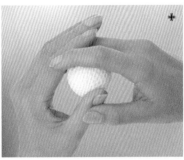

Rest a golf ball in the BRAIN reflex area, and then roll the ball through the area for several minutes.

Dizziness & fever

Work the pituitary gland reflex area to help ease these health concerns. When experiencing dizziness (or fainting), apply technique until the feeling subsides. If, however, you are trying to reduce a fever, work the pituitary gland reflex area every hour.

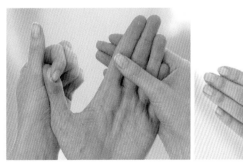

Rest your fingertip on the PITUITARY GLAND reflex area. Press gently several times.

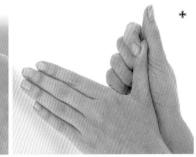

Find the PITUITARY GLAND reflex area on your fingertip, and then press the spot gently several times.

Stomachache

For a stomachache apply technique to the stomach reflex area until discomfort diminishes. If you are prone to having an upset stomach, work this reflex area several times a day as a preventive measure.

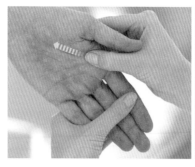

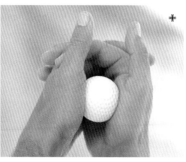

Hold the hand steady and thumb-walk throughout the STOMACH reflex area, making several passes.

Rest a golf ball between your hands. Roll it throughout the STOMACH reflex area.

Heartburn & hiatal hernia

To target heartburn and hiatal hernia concerns, work the solar plexus reflex area for several minutes 3–4 times a day. As you apply the thumb-walking or golf ball technique, concentrate on any sensitive areas.

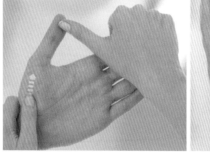

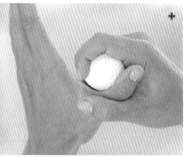

Hold the hand up as shown and thumb-walk around the base of the thumb in successive passes.

Grip a golf ball in your fingers. Now, rest it at the base of the thumb and roll it around the area.

Diarrhea & diverticulitis

For these conditions, apply reflexology to the colon reflex area for several minutes, 3–4 times a day. This can also help ease the symptoms of colitis.

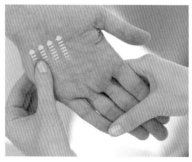

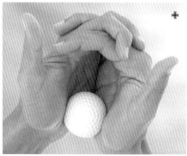

Work the COLON reflex area, making a succession of thumb-walking passes throughout the area.

Roll a golf ball through the COLON reflex area for several minutes. Repeat 3–4 times a day.

Diabetes & hypoglycemia (low blood sugar)

In some forms of diabetes the pancreas secretes too little insulin, a hormone that helps to metabolize sugar. For diabetes and hypoglycemia, work the pancreas reflex area and then the kidney reflex area to help eliminate toxins. Note: do not overwork the pancreas reflex area – apply pressure gently and briefly.

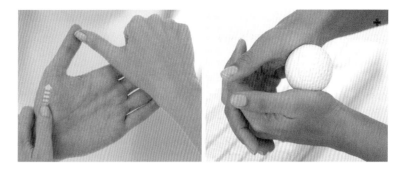

Holding the hand in place, thumb-walk several times throughout the PANCREAS reflex area.

Rest a golf ball between your hands, and roll it through the KIDNEY and PANCREAS reflex areas several times.

Menstrual cramps & PMS

To help relieve the discomfort of menstrual cramps or premenstrual syndrome (PMS), target the uterus reflex area. Apply technique to the area until discomfort subsides. If you are prone to PMS, work this reflex area several times a day as a preventive measure.

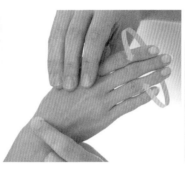

Rest your fingertip on the UTERUS reflex area and rotate the hand several times in both directions.

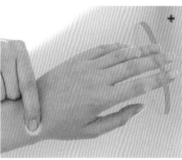

Place your fingertip on the UTERUS reflex area and rotate your wrist several times in both directions.

Insomnia

Tension is usually the culprit if you have trouble falling asleep and staying asleep. Use reflexology just before bedtime to relax. Apply technique to the solar plexus and neck reflex areas. Follow these exercises with a relaxing series of desserts (*see pages 60–65 and 82–85*).

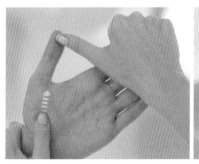

Hold the hand in place and repeatedly thumb-walk through the SOLAR PLEXUS reflex area.

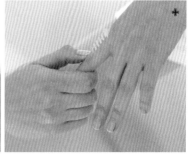

Apply the walk-down/pull-against to each digit to work the NECK reflex area, making several passes.

USING REFLEXOLOGY FOR HAND CONCERNS

Using reflexology to deal with specifically hand-related problems involves many of the same techniques and concepts as are applied to deal with problems in other parts of the body. In this section, we explain how to choose techniques that are best suited to dealing with your hand concerns, detailing how much, how long, and how often to apply them. We explain the use of pressure, stretch, movement, and other sensory experiences to help relieve hand problems. In addition, we'll consider your hand profile.

Many different types of job subject the hands to excessive demands, which can result in strain and injury. Manual workers, for example, may develop problems as a result of lifting heavy weights, from the constant vibration of power tools, or from the repetitive patterns of movement involved in using other tools and equipment. Office workers, on the other hand, may

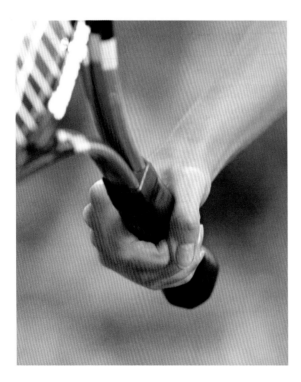

suffer from carpal tunnel syndrome or repetitive stress injury (RSI) – both types of hand injury that may result from the repetitive movements of keyboard use.

WHY HANDS ARE IMPORTANT

Whatever the source of potential problems, maintenance of the hands' abilities is crucial for quality of life. The ability to use one's hands is of paramount importance in many jobs and lifestyles, with injury or strain potentially inhibiting not just work but also the things you enjoy doing in your spare time, such as sports or knitting or playing a musical instrument.

In addition to such obvious hand concerns, a hand problem may, according to reflexology theory, reflect or create a health concern. What started out as a hand stress can become a stress on the body (and vice versa). An injured finger, for example, may affect the neck, since the finger reflects the neck reflex area. Moreover, the neck is the source of muscles and nerves that create movement of the fingers, so any change in the finger's capabilities changes the actions of the arm and neck. All the more reason to keep your hands happy, since their health is so closely linked to your general well-being.

Overuse of the hands in sports, such as tennis, may give rise to strain or injury. Conversely, hand injuries may curtail participation in sports and other hobbies.

CAUTIONS

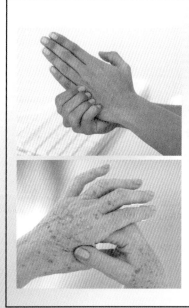

When working with a hand that is injured or aching, certain precautions must be observed:

Never work directly on an injury or an area that is sore to the touch. If you work on such a hand, set up clear boundaries to the work that can be done. If necessary, avoid working on the hand altogether.

Don't try to place too much stress on an already stressed hand. When overdone, the workout can be taxing instead of relaxing. Always be sure to work within the individual's comfort zone.

When working with older hands, be careful not to overwork, especially by applying too many hand desserts. Just as overworking muscles can have uncomfortable results, so overmoving a hand can also result in pain or discomfort.

Don't try to be too ambitious or expect instant results. If your hand problem has taken time to develop, it will take a while to bring about relief.

TIPS FOR ADDRESSING HAND CONCERNS

First, consider why your hands are tired or in pain. Aside from injury or arthritis, what it is that you do and possibly overdo with your hands? Think about your work, sports, hobbies, and volunteer activities. How often and for how long do you tax your hands?

Make it a rule to work and play only within the limits of your hands' comfort. Watch what you do with your hands: they are not hammers, wrenches, or pliers. Also, think before you act. For example, 60 percent of hand injuries at work would be avoided if workers wore gloves. When you put your hands to work, use them wisely.

Think about relaxation: how much, how long, and how often do you relax your hands?

Interrupt stress and do it frequently. Try this experiment: apply relaxation technique morning, noon, and night; or, pay attention to your hands each time they feel stressed. Figure out your pattern; discover which techniques can keep your hands happy. If your strategy is not working, try something else, a different technique, or maybe applying it at a different time of day.

KEYBOARDING

From computers to electronic gadgets and games, it seems that hands don't have a moment's rest in our technological world. Overuse of a computer keyboard can bring about carpal tunnel-like symptoms (*see pages 148–149*), while using the mini-keyboards on cellular phones and electronic games overtaxes the thumb. The relaxation exercises below can offer hands some relief.

Working the hands

The thumb plays a role in 50 percent of the hand's activities, and tension accumulated in the thumb can radiate outward to affect the whole hand. The following relaxation technique will help to reduce the strain. Once you've worked the hand in the four directions described, consider which movement showed the most stress.

1 Rest your hand in the palm of the hand to be worked. Press down gently with the heel of your hand. Hold for several seconds.

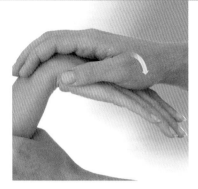

2 Press down gently on the top of the hand with the heel of your hand; hold for several seconds.

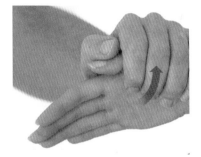

3 Rest your palm on top of the hand and curl your fingers around the edge of the hand. Gently pull up with your fingers.

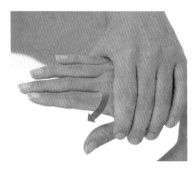

4 Now curl your thumb around the other edge of the hand and pull upward, while pressing down with your fingers. Hold for several seconds.

Working a self-help strategy

A self-help strategy works well when you need a break for your tired hands. Rolling a golf ball around between the hands works several reflex areas, and is a useful self-help tool (*see pages 102–109*).

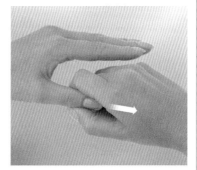

Relaxation techniques

The repetitive nature of typing at a keyboard can lead to tense, tired hands. One of the best ways to break up these habitual stress patterns is use the directional-movement stretches (*see below and page 47*). The complete range of movement this self-help exercise provides helps to relax the hands.

KEEPING THUMBS HAPPY

Text messaging and electronic games have introduced a new type of challenge for the thumb. Keep your thumbs happy by reducing the demands on them, resting them between bouts of use, and applying compensatory techniques. Pay attention to all the activities that place a strain on your thumb, considering the time you spent on different activities and their impact.

1 Gently pull your thumb. Turn it in first a clockwise and then a counter-clockwise direction. Repeat on each digit in turn.

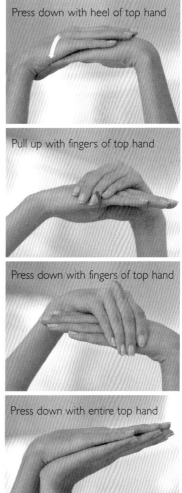

Press down with heel of top hand

Pull up with fingers of top hand

Press down with fingers of top hand

Press down with entire top hand

2 Now, go on to apply side-to-side movement to each finger. Rest your fingers around the finger. Gently move the joint from side to side. Go on to each finger.

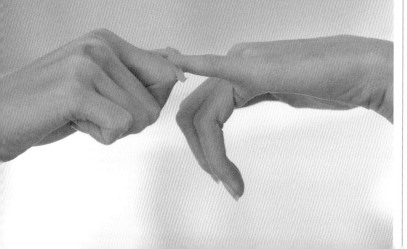

SPORTING HANDS

Participation in sports can place heavy demands on the hands – from the "handlebar palsy" suffered by cyclists who lean too heavily on their handlebars to the type of thumb injury that skiers commonly sustain. Whatever your sport, be aware of the strains being placed on your hands, adjusting your technique if necessary, and resting the hands when injury or strain occurs.

> ### CAUTION
> Always seek medical advice for any injury and follow the physician's recommendations. Rest is always best when it comes to strain-related injuries, so give your hand a chance to recover. Take care not to overstretch an injured hand, and never apply reflexology techniques directly to an injury.

Working the hands

As you apply these techniques, try to pinpoint areas of strain and overuse. For injured hands, however, seek a medical opinion before proceeding with your work.

CARE FOR SPORTY HANDS

When engaging in any sporting activity, always wear the appropriate protective gloves or mitts to protect your hands.

Know when enough is enough. If your hand is constantly aching following your nightly handball game, take some time off.

Consider adopting a warm-up or cool-down routine for your hands. Add some basic stretches, or try using health balls (see page 44) to strengthen your hands.

Between sessions, apply hand relaxation techniques, concentrating on overused parts of the hand.

When working with others, be sensitive to the individual. Be aware of his or her comfort zone.

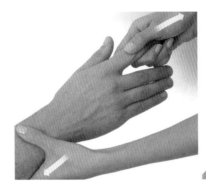

1 Hold the hand steady at the wrist and apply a finger-pull to each digit, simultaneously pulling gently and slowly in both directions.

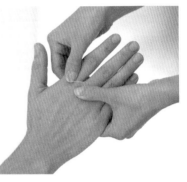

2 Hold the hand as shown. Alternately and rhythmically pull and push with the flats of the thumbs. Repeat several times.

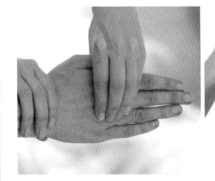

3 Hold the hand at the wrist. Press gently on the long bone of each finger several times.

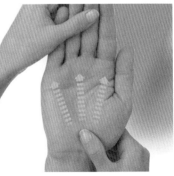

4 Holding the hand upright, make a series of thumb-walking passes throughout the palm

Self-help hand reflexology

As you apply these self-help reflexology techniques, think about what feels good and what doesn't, so that you become aware of your hands' tension levels. If you have suffered a hand injury, allow it time to recover before starting to apply technique.

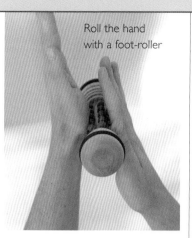

Roll the hand with a foot-roller

Relaxation techniques

For hands that have become over-stressed through sporting activities, the application of self-help techniques can help overall hand relaxation. In addition, these techniques can improve the hand's range of movement. This increased flexibility and relaxation, can not only help to speed recovery, but also to prevent future injury.

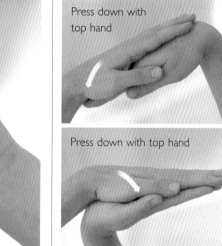

1 Grasp a finger and pull slowly. Hold for several seconds. Now turn the finger clockwise and counter-clockwise. Repeat on each finger and thumb in turn.

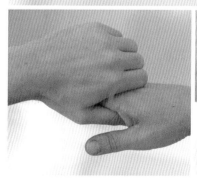

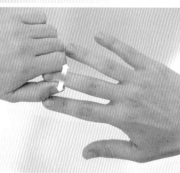

2 Clasping the hand as shown, repeatedly push down on the knuckle above the middle finger.

3 Hold the finger as shown and apply the side-to-side technique. Repeat on each joint of each digit.

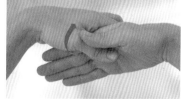

Press down with top hand

Press down with top hand

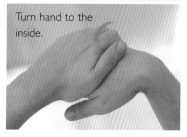

Turn hand to the outside

Turn hand to the inside.

TIRED & SORE HANDS

If your hands are tired and sore, think about what caused the problem and seek ways of avoiding such stress in the future. Using self-help techniques may tire your hands even more, but a warm paraffin-wax bath is soothing and requires very little effort. Alternatively, ask a friend to apply the following desserts.

Working the hands

When working on someone with tired or sore hands, be aware of his or her comfort level. Focus on relaxing the hands by applying lots of desserts. Slowly and gently apply the techniques listed below.

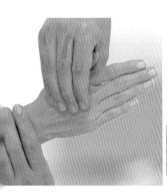

1 Repeatedly press down on the back of the hand as shown.

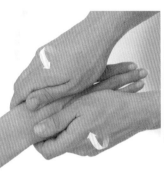

2 Grasp the recipient's hand as shown, and stretch the hand outward.

3 Apply the side-to-side technique to each joint of each digit in turn.

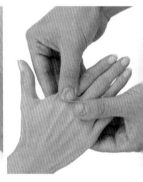

4 Move and counter-move the long bones as shown.

5 Grasp each digit and apply the squeeze technique, holding for several seconds. Finish by applying the squeeze to the whole hand. Repeat on both hands.

Working with a self-help strategy

While you are always the best judge of how and when to soothe your own tired or sore hands, the tips below can help.

1 If your hands are tired and aching, you'll want to begin your work with techniques that require minimal effort. Try a paraffin-wax bath or massaging the hand with a wand vibrator. Both offer soothing, general relaxation with very little effort.

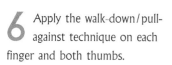

6 Apply the walk-down/pull-against technique on each finger and both thumbs.

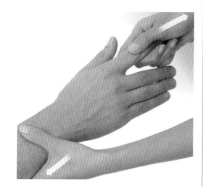

7 Gently apply the finger-pull technique to each finger and thumb in turn.

HELPING TIRED HANDS

Consider what you overdo and either eliminate the activity or compensate with a counter-movement. For example, after curling your fingers around a tennis racket for lengthy periods, stretch them in the opposite direction to relax them.

Use TV-viewing time to relax your hands with a vibrating wand.

Think about your hands before launching into a project. If they are tired and sore, avoid activities that will cause further stress.

2 When your hands are tired or sore, think about which part is most stressed and focus your effort there. For example, if you have an overstressed thumb, hold it as you watch television, gently stretching and rubbing. The goal is maximum relaxation with minimal effort.

3 Focus on what you find most relaxing for your hands and your body. Once you've identified your favorites, stick with them.

CARPAL TUNNEL SYNDROME

Carpal tunnel syndrome is a repetitive strain injury resulting from compression of the median nerve at the wrist. Symptoms include pain, numbness, and tingling in the fingers, hands, and forearms. In some cases, the condition is associated with occupations that involve repetitive hand movements, such as keyboarding. The following techniques will help to relax the hand and may reduce the symptoms.

Working the hands

Before you begin work, review with the recipient which directions of movement or parts of the hand are particularly sensitive.

2 Thumb-walk lightly between the heels of the hand (the impacted median nerve is in the area between the two heels of the hand).

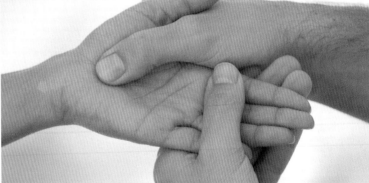

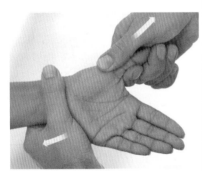

1 Pull gently on the thumb with one hand, while stretching the hand back with the other.

3 Holding the hand as shown, press down with the fingers while pushing up with the thumb.

DOS AND DON'TS

Start out gently, maintaining eye contact as you work to check that you are causing no pain. Be aware of how long you have worked.

Don't overwork the hand or work too long. Be careful not to pull too hard on the fingers, or to overly turn the hand.

Working with self-help techniques

Tendon glides help to alleviate the symptoms associated with carpal tunnel syndrome by stretching and strengthening under-used muscles. Repeat the following sequence 3–5 times to begin with, gradually building up to 10 cycles.

Tendon glides

1 Hold your hand upright with your fingers and thumb outstretched.

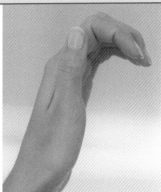

2 Make a hook with your fingers by curling them inward. Keep the thumb straight.

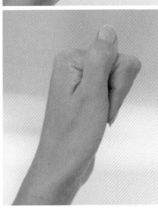

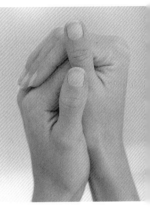

3 Curl your fingers over to touch your palm. Now curl your thumb over your fingers to make a fist and squeeze.

4 Wrap your other hand around your fist and squeeze. Repeat the entire sequence several times.

The squeeze

To further relax the hands, apply the squeeze technique on each hand. Repeat several times.

ARTHRITIS

Arthritis is a painful condition involving inflammation of the joints. Since arthritis affects the whole body, aim to work the whole hand, applying desserts to encourage a better range of motion. Work the kidney reflex areas to help eliminate waste products from the body, and the adrenal gland reflex areas to help fight inflammation, a characteristic of arthritis. Targeting the solar plexus reflex area can relieve tension, which is a contributory factor in arthritis.

RESEARCH
Researchers in China found that reflexology can ease the pain of arthritis. Results from the same study suggest that the application of self-help reflexology techniques can help to maintain these results. Other research has found that reflexology can help ease stiffness in the joints as well as the pain associated with it.

Working the hands

When working on someone with arthritic hands, be gentle and ensure that you work within his or her comfort zone.

1 To encourage better flexibility, apply some desserts. Grasp the index finger and pull gently. Repeat on each digit on both hands.

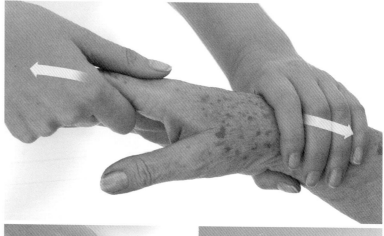

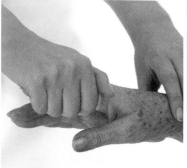

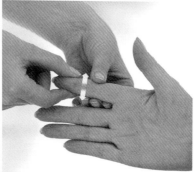

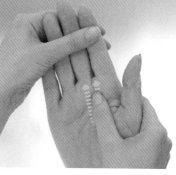

2 Gently squeeze the base of the finger and repeat along the entire length of the finger. Repeat the dessert on each digit.

3 Apply the finger side-to-side dessert to the joints of each finger and thumb, being careful not to use too much force.

4 For a calming effect, thumb-walk lightly throughout the SOLAR PLEXUS reflex area, making several successive passes.

POINTS TO REMEMBER

Self-help hand reflexology

Applying reflexology to the hands for arthritis involves two strategies: one is to work the reflex areas associated with the overall condition and the other is to use desserts to encourage movement of stiff joints.

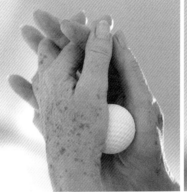

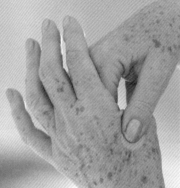

1 Begin by rolling a golf ball over the ADRENAL GLAND reflex area, the general area in the heel of the hand below the thumb.

2 Now, press gently into the KIDNEY reflex area located deep in the webbing of the thumb and index finger. Hold for a few seconds.

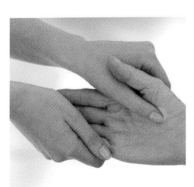

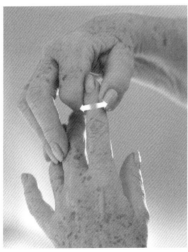

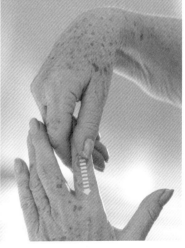

5 With the thumb, press into the KIDNEY reflex area on the webbing and hold for several seconds. Reposition and press again.

3 Mobilize stiff joints by applying the finger side-to-side dessert. Work the joints of each digit.

4 To maintain flexibility, apply the walk-down/pull-against dessert to each of the fingers and the thumb.

HAND INJURY

Accidents happen and, since hands are crucial to so many jobs, it's not surprising that hand injury is a common occurrence, making up one-third of all traumatic injuries. For serious injuries, especially those involving deep cuts, burns, or possible fractures, seek medical advice. But for minor injuries, the following exercises can help to relax the hand, easing the pain, and aiding your recovery.

Working the hands

Injured hands require a light touch. Ask the recipient which part of the hand is painful and then aim to work around it.

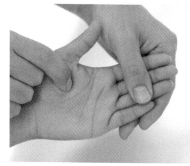

LEARNING TIP

Always move slowly and cautiously when working with a hand that has been injured: failure to do so may delay its recovery. Whatever you do, try not to be overly ambitious. This means you should avoid working the hand for too long, or moving it too rapidly.

---

1 With the tip of the index finger, apply light pressure to the palm of the hand, avoiding direct contact with any injury.

2 Once the pain has subsided a little, thumb-walk lightly through the palm of the hand.

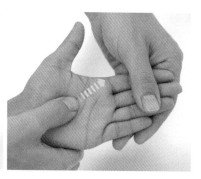

3 Apply the finger-pull dessert to relax the whole hand, gently pulling each digit.

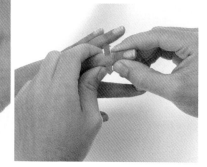

4 The finger side-to-side dessert relaxes the digits. Gently move the finger joint from side to side, as shown. Repeat on each finger and thumb in turn.

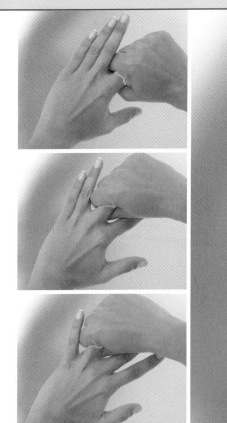

Working with self-help techniques

Injury can strike at any time, which makes self-help techniques all the more important. Try the techniques below to help ease the pain of injury.

1 Begin by gently squeezing the injured part of your hand. Then reposition your hand and squeeze along the length of the hand from wrist to fingertips.

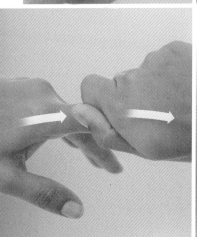

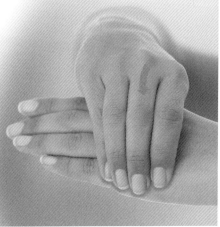

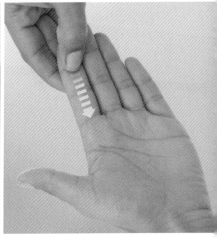

2 Gently apply the finger-pull technique to each finger and thumb in turn, enclosing the digit within the right hand. Continue until the hand feels relaxed.

3 Rest the working fingers on the top of the hand, with the working thumb underneath, on the palm. Push upward with the thumb as you press down with the fingers.

4 Thumb-walk gently across the area that is recovering from injury. The picture above shows an injured index finger being worked on.

RESOURCES

Finding a reflexologist

If you decide to visit a professional reflexologist instead of or in addition to self-application of reflexology techniques at home, check the practitioner's credentials for any qualifications and membership of reflexology organizations (*see below*). Bear in mind, however, that standards have changed over the past decade, so check with prospective practitioners the date and duration of their study, and how much professional experience they have had since qualifying. The best-qualified reflexologists have completed a course of study of 50 hours or more, followed by at least a year's experience. It is worth noting that someone who has expanded into other areas (such as selling products or other complementary therapies) may not be as experienced in reflexology as a specialist.

Contacts

Australia

Reflexology Association of Australia
P.O. Box 366, Cammeray, NSW 2062
Web: www.raansw.com.au

International Council
of Reflexologists
P.O. Box 1032, Bondi Junction
NSW
Phone: 61 612 9300 9391

Canada

Reflexology Association of
British Columbia
#214-3707 Hamber Place
N. Vancouver
British Columbia
V7G 2J4
www.reflexologybc.com

Reflexology Association of
Canada
P.O. Box 1605, Station Main
Winnipeg, Manitoba
www.reflexologycanada.ca

Reflexology Registration Council
of Ontario
P. O. Box 6
Palgrave, Ontario L0N 1P0
Email: info@rrco-reflexology.com

International Council
of Reflexologists
P. O. Box 78060
Westcliffe Postal Outlet
Hamilton, Ontario L9C 7N5
www.icr-reflexology.org

New Zealand

The New Zealand Institute
of Reflexologists Inc.
253 Mount Albert Road,
Mount Roskill
Auckland

New Zealand Reflexology
Association
P.O. Box 31 084
Auckland 9
Phone: 64 9 486 1918

Republic of Ireland

Irish Reflexologists' Institute
1 St Anne's Cottages,
Gold Links Road
Bettystown, Co. Meath
Email: editor@reflexology.ie

National Register of Reflexologists
(Ireland)
Unit 13, Upper Mall
Terryland Retail Park
Headford Road, Galway
Phone: 353 91 568844

United Kingdom

Association of Reflexologists
27 Old Gloucester Street
London, WC1N 3XX
Email: aor@reflexology.org

British Reflexology Association
Monks Orchard,
Whitbourne
Worcester, WR6 5RB
Web: www.britreflex.co.uk

International Federation
of Reflexologists
78 Edridge Road
Croydon
Surrey, CRO 1EF
Phone: 0208 645 9134

International Institute
of Reflexology (UK)
255 Turleigh
Bradford-on-Avon
Wiltshire, BA15 2HG
Phone: 01225 865899

United States

**New York State Reflexology
Association**
142 E. 23rd St., Suite 4
NY, NY 10010
www.newyorkstatereflexology.org

**Pennsylvania Reflexology
Association**
P.O. Box 233
Hellertown, PA 18055

**Reflexology Association of
America**
4012 S. Rainbow Blvd.
K-Box PMB #585
Las Vegas, NV 89103

**Washington Reflexology
Association**
www.washingtonreflexology.org

Websites

www.reflexology-research.com
Kevin and Barbara Kunz's website;
offers the basics on reflexology
theory, practice, and research.

www.foot-reflexologist.com
Kevin and Barbara Kunz offer
information and advice for
professional reflexologists.

www.reflexology.org
Links to important reflexology
websites, and list of worldwide
reflexology organizations.

www.iol.ie / ~footman / booklst.html
Lists useful reflexology books,
videos, and charts, and where to
purchase them.

Further reading

Gillanders, Ann
Reflexology: A Step-by-Step Guide
(Element Books, 1997)

Hall, Nicola
Reflexology: A Way to Better Health
(Newleaf, 2001)

Kunz, Kevin and Barbara
*Reflexology: Health at your
Fingertips*
(Dorling Kindersley, 2003)

Kunz, Kevin and Barbara
My Reflexologist Says Feet Don't Lie
(Reflexology Research Project Press,
2001)

Kunz, Kevin and Barbara
Hand Reflexology Workbook (Revised)
(Reflexology Research Project Press,
1999)

Kunz, Kevin and Barbara
*The Complete Guide to Foot
Reflexology (Revised)*
(Reflexology Research Project Press,
2005)

Kunz, Kevin and Barbara
*Hand and Foot Reflexology:
A Self-Help Guide*
(Simon & Schuster, 1992)

Lett, Anne
*Reflex Zone Therapy for Healthcare
Professionals*
(Churchill Livingstone, 2000)

Marquardt, Hanne
Reflex Zone Therapy of the Feet
(Inner Traditions Intl Ltd, 1996)

Eugster, Father Josef
*The Rwo Shur Health Method:
A Self Study Book on Foot
Reflexology*
(Geraldine Co., 1988)

INDEX

A

abdominal pain 130, 131
adrenal gland reflex area 122
  allergies & hay fever 135
  anxiety & depression 136
  arthritis 151
  asthma 134
  breast cancer recovery 132, 133
  children 111
  commuters 117
  golf-ball sequence 103, 108
  heart problems 136
  high blood pressure 135
  left hand sequences 68, 69, 88, 89
  low energy & fatigue 134
  maps 16, 17
  pregnant women 113
  right hand sequences 79, 98
  sinus problems & headaches 135
  stress reduction 124, 125
  travelers 119
adrenaline 13, 122, 134, 136
allergies 135
anatomy 38–9
anxiety & depression 136
arm reflex area
  left hand sequences 72, 73, 92, 93
  maps 16, 17
  right hand sequences 81, 101
arthritis 150–1
asthma 134

B

babies 26, 32, 110, 123
back reflex areas see specific areas
  (e.g. upper back reflex area)
backache & neck pain 113, 128–9
balls 44, 144
  see also golf balls
baths, paraffin-wax 53, 147, 151
benefits 6, 13, 21–33
  see also specific benefits (e.g. relaxation)
bladder reflex area, maps 16, 17
blood sugar levels 123, 134, 139
bone marrow 38
bones 38–9
brain reflex area
  golf-ball sequence 102, 107, 109
  headaches 126
  heart problems 136
  incontinence 136

left hand sequences 66, 67, 74, 75, 86, 87, 94, 95
  maps 16, 17
  right hand sequences 78, 79, 80, 99, 101
  stroke 137
breast cancer recovery 132–3
breast reflex area
  breast cancer recovery 132, 133
  golf-ball sequence 104, 109
  left hand sequences 76, 77, 96, 97
  maps 18, 19
  right hand sequences 80, 81, 100
brittle nails 39

C

carpal tunnel syndrome 27, 41, 140, 142, 148–9
carpals 38, 39
case studies 32–3
charts 14–19
chest pain 130, 131
chest reflex area
  breast cancer recovery 132, 133
  golf-ball sequence 104, 109
  left hand sequences 70, 71, 76, 77, 90, 91, 96, 97
  maps 16 -19
  right hand sequences 79, 80, 81, 99, 100
children 27, 32, 111, 123
colic in babies 110
colon reflex area
  babies 110
  diarrhea & diverticulitis 138
  digestive problems 28, 110, 138
  elderly people 28
  golf-ball sequence 105, 109
  left hand sequences 72, 73, 92, 93
  pregnant women 113
  right hand sequences 80, 101
color, fingernails 39
comfort zone 52, 123, 141, 150, 151
communication skills 51, 52
commuters 116–17
cramps & PMS 139
cupping 45

D

depression 28, 30, 136
desserts
  arthritis 150, 151
  breast cancer recovery 133

elderly people 28
  golf-ball sequence 108–9
  left hand self-help sequence 86, 87, 89, 91, 93, 95, 97
  left hand sequence 66, 67, 69, 71, 73, 75, 77
  office workers & keyboarders 27, 115, 143
  right hand sequences 78–81, 98–101, 108–9
  self-help 82–5
  techniques 60–5, 82–5
  tired & sore hands 146–7
diabetes & hypoglycemia 123, 134, 139
diaphragm, lateral marker 14, 15
diaphragm reflex area
  left hand self-help sequence 88, 89, 90, 91, 92, 93
  left hand sequence 68, 69, 70, 71, 72, 73
  maps 16–19
  right hand sequence 81
diarrhea 110, 138
digestive problems 28, 110, 118, 122, 138
directional movement stretches 47, 118, 142, 143
diverticulitis 138
dizziness & fever 137

E

ear reflex area
  babies 110
  left hand sequences 70, 71, 90, 91
  maps 16, 17
  right hand sequences 80, 100
elderly people 23, 27, 28, 30, 31, 123
equipment see tools
ergonomics 40–1
esophagus reflex area, babies 110
eye reflex area
  left hand sequences 70, 71, 90, 91
  maps 16, 17
  right hand sequences 79, 99

F

face reflex area, headaches 126
fainting, dizziness & fever 137
fallopian tubes reflex area
  left hand sequences 76, 77, 96, 97
  maps 18, 19
  right hand sequences 80, 101
FAQs 23, 25, 35

fatigue & low energy 134
fever & dizziness 137
finger side-to-side
　arthritis 150, 151
　backache & neck pain 128, 129
　commuters 117
　golf-ball sequence 109
　hand injuries 153
　left hand sequences 66, 86, 87
　office workers & keyboarders 115, 143
　right hand sequences 78, 98, 99, 100, 109
　sinus problems & headaches 135
　sporting hands 145
　techniques 63, 83
　tired & sore hands 146
finger-pull
　arthritis 150
　children 111
　commuters 116
　elderly people 28
　golf-ball sequence 109
　hand injuries 152, 153
　left hand sequences 66, 67, 69, 73, 75, 77, 86, 89, 93
　office workers & keyboarders 115, 143
　pregnant women 112
　right hand sequences 78, 80, 81, 98, 99, 100, 109
　sporting hands 144, 145
　techniques 63, 82
　tired & sore hands 147
finger-walking 56–7
fingernails 39, 50, 107
　see also nail-buffing
fluid retention 137
foot reflexology 24, 25

G

gall bladder reflex area 17, 73, 93, 101, 105, 109
gloves 43, 141, 144
golf balls & golf-ball techniques
　health concerns see specific health concerns (e.g headaches)
　office workers & keyboarders 27, 114, 143
　overuse risk 23
　pregnant women 32, 113
　self-help sequence 102–9
gripping 45
groin reflex area
　left hand sequences 76, 77, 96, 97
　maps 18, 19
　right hand sequences 80, 101

gums reflex area
　left hand sequences 74, 75, 86, 94, 95
　maps 18, 19
　right hand sequences 80, 99, 101

H

hand-stretcher 60
　left hand sequence 66, 69, 73, 75
　right hand sequence 79, 80, 81
hands
　hand anatomy 38–9
　hand care 37–47
　hand concerns 140–53
　hand courtesy 51
　hand injuries 152–3
　hand maps 14–19
　hand spas 13
　importance 12, 13, 140
　session preparation 50
hay fever 6, 135
head pain 130, 131
　headaches 126–7, 135
head reflex area
　golf-ball sequence 102, 107, 109
　headaches 126, 127
　left hand sequences 66, 67, 74, 75, 86, 87, 94, 95
　maps 16–19
　office workers & keyboarders 115
　pain 130, 131
　right hand sequences 78, 79, 80, 99, 101
headaches 126–7, 135
health balls 44, 144
health concerns 6, 13, 21–33, 52, 122–3
　see also specific concerns (e.g. headaches)
heart problems 136
heart reflex area
　golf-ball sequence 102, 104
　heart problems 136
　left hand sequences 70, 71, 90, 91
　maps 16, 17
　right hand sequences 79, 98
heartburn & hiatal hernia 138
high blood pressure 135
hip reflex area 18, 19, 76, 80, 129
history 10–11
hook & back-up 58, 119, 126
hospital & hospice patients 28, 30
hypoglycemia & diabetes 123, 134, 139

I

incontinence 136
inflammation 135, 150
injuries 40–1, 140, 144, 152–3

prevention & safety 43, 113, 123, 140, 141
　see also specific problems (e.g. carpal tunnel syndrome)
inner ear reflex area
　left hand sequences 70, 71, 90, 91
　maps 16, 17
　right hand sequences 80, 99
insomnia 139

J

jaw reflex area
　left hand sequences 74, 75, 86, 94, 95
　maps 18, 19
　right hand sequences 80, 99, 101

K

keyboarding & office work
　ergonomics 40–1
　self-help 27, 114–15, 142–3
　warm-up/relaxation exercises 43, 46–7, 143
kidney reflex area
　arthritis 151
　diabetes & hypoglycemia 139
　fluid retention 137
　golf-ball sequence 103, 108
　left hand sequences 68, 69, 88, 89
　maps 16, 17
　pregnant women 113
　right hand sequences 78, 79, 99
knee reflex area 18, 19, 76, 80, 129

L

lateral markers 14–15
left hand maps 15, 16, 18
left hand sequences 66–77, 86–97, 102–7
leg reflex area 18, 19
leverage 104
liver reflex area 17, 73, 101, 105, 109
low blood sugar see diabetes & hypoglycemia
low energy & fatigue 134
lower back reflex area
　backache & neck pain 129
　golf-ball sequence 105, 109
　left hand sequences 73, 76, 77, 96, 97
　maps 16–19
　pregnant women 113
　right hand sequences 80, 100
lung reflex area
　breast cancer recovery 132, 133
　golf-ball sequence 104, 109
　left hand sequences 70, 71, 76, 77, 90, 91, 96, 97

maps 16–19
right hand sequences 79, 80, 81, 99, 100
lymph glands reflex area
breast cancer recovery 132, 133
left hand sequences 76, 77, 96, 97
maps 18, 19
right hand sequences 80, 101

M

maps 14–19
median nerve compression 41, 148
medical care 6, 26–33, 52, 122–3
see also specific health concerns (e.g. headaches)
menstrual cramps & PMS 139
metacarpals 38, 39
migraine headaches 127
multiple finger-walking 57, 114, 128, 129
muscles 38

N

nail-buffing
golf-ball sequence 109
self-help sequence 86, 95, 99, 101
technique 84
nails 39, 50, 107
neck
base of neck lateral marker 14, 15
pain 128–9, 130, 131
neck reflex area
backache & neck pain 128, 129
commuters 116, 117
golf-ball sequence 102, 106, 108, 109
headaches 126, 127
insomnia 139
left hand sequences 66, 67, 74, 75, 86, 87, 94, 95
maps 16–19
pain 130, 131
right hand sequences 78, 79, 80, 99, 101

O

office work see keyboarding & office work
older people 23, 27, 28, 30, 31, 123
ovary/testicle reflex area
left hand sequences 76, 77, 96, 97
maps 18, 19
right hand sequences 80, 101
overuse 23, 140, 144

P

pain 130–1
see also specific pains (e.g. headaches)

palm counter-mover
commuters 117
golf-ball sequence 108
left hand sequences 66, 71, 86, 91
pregnant women 113
right hand sequences 79, 98, 100, 101, 108
techniques 62, 85
palm-mover
carpal tunnel syndrome 148
commuters 117
golf-ball sequence 108
hand injuries 153
left hand sequences 66, 71, 86, 91
right hand sequences 79, 80, 81, 98, 100, 101, 108
techniques 62, 85
travelers 119
palm-rocker
left hand sequence 66, 67, 69, 71, 73, 77
right hand sequence 78, 79, 81
technique 61
palms
golf-ball sequence 104, 105
left hand sequences 70–3, 90–3
palm maps 15, 16–17
right hand sequences 78–81, 98–101
pancreas reflex area
anxiety & depression 136
children 111
diabetes & hypoglycemia 123, 134, 139
golf-ball sequence 103, 108
left hand sequences 68, 69, 88, 89
low energy & fatigue 134
maps 16, 17
office workers & keyboarders 114
pregnant women 113
right hand sequences 79, 99
travelers 119
paraffin-wax baths 53, 147, 151
parathyroid gland reflex area
golf-ball sequence 102, 109
left hand sequences 66, 86, 87
maps 16–19
right hand sequences 79, 99
phalanges 38, 39
physical disabilities 28
pituitary gland reflex area
children 111
dizziness & fever 137
left hand sequences 66, 67, 86, 87
maps 16, 17
right hand sequences 79, 99
PMS & menstrual cramps 139
post-natal depression 28, 30

practitioners, assessing 34–5
pregnant women 28, 30, 32, 112–13, 123
preparation & timing, reflexology sessions 50–3
pressing 45
pressure sensors 13
prostate gland see uterus/prostate gland reflex area

R

reflex areas
see specific areas (e.g. neck reflex area)
reflexologists, assessing 34–5
reflexology sessions
golf-ball sequence 102–9
left hand sequences 66–77, 86–97
preparation & timing 50–3
right hand sequences 78–81, 98–101
relaxation 27, 53, 141
anxiety & depression 136
breast cancer recovery 133
office workers & keyboarders 43, 46–7, 142–3, 149
pregnant women 112, 113
relaxation response 13
sporting hands 145
tension relief 130, 131, 139
repetitive stress injuries 40–1, 140
see also specific problems (eg carpal tunnel syndrome)
research studies 13, 29, 30–1, 124, 126, 128, 130, 132, 150
ridged nails 39
right hand maps 15, 17, 19
right hand sequences 78–81, 98–101, 108–9
rollers 44, 53, 145
rotating on a point 59

S

safety & injury prevention 43, 113, 123, 140, 141
self-help
commuters 116–17
desserts 82–5
efficacy 25, 31
elderly people 31
golf-ball sequence 102–9
health concerns see specific health concerns (e.g. headaches)
left hand sequence 86–97
office workers & keyboarders 27, 114–15, 142–3
pregnant women 113
right hand sequence 98–101

sporting hands 145
tired & sore hands 147
tools 23, 44–5, 50, 51, 53, 145, 147, 151
travelers 118–19
see also golf balls & golf-ball techniques
sessions see reflexology sessions
shoulder reflex area
golf-ball sequence 104, 108
left hand sequences 70, 71, 90, 91
maps 16–19
office workers & keyboarders 115
right hand sequences 79, 99
sinus problems & headaches 135
sinus reflex area
golf-ball sequence 102, 107, 109
headaches 126
left hand sequences 66, 67, 74, 75, 86,
87, 94, 95
maps 16–19
right hand sequences 78, 79, 80, 99, 101
skin care 43
small intestine reflex area
golf-ball sequence 105, 109
left hand sequences 72, 73, 92, 93
maps 16, 17
right hand sequences 80, 101
solar plexus reflex area
anxiety & depression 136
arthritis 150
babies 110
breast cancer recovery 132, 133
children 111
commuters 116
heartburn & hiatal hernia 138
high blood pressure 135
insomnia 139
left hand sequence 68, 69
maps 16–19
office workers & keyboarders 115
pain 130, 131
pregnant women 112, 113
right hand sequence 78, 79
stress reduction 124, 125
travelers 119
sore & tired hands 146–7
spine reflex area
backache & neck pain 128, 129
children 111
golf-ball sequence 106, 108
left hand sequences 74, 75, 94, 95
maps 16–19
migraine headaches 127
right hand sequences 81, 100, 101
spleen reflex area 16, 73, 105, 109
sporting hands 144–5

spots on nails 39
squeeze
carpal tunnel syndrome 149
elderly people 28
golf-ball sequence 108
hand injuries 153
left hand self-help sequence 86, 89
pregnant women 112
right hand self-help sequence 98, 101
techniques 65, 85
tired & sore hands 146
stomach reflex area
golf-ball sequence 103, 105, 108, 109
left hand self-help sequence 88, 89, 90,
91, 92, 93
left hand sequence 68, 69, 72, 73
maps 16, 17
right hand sequence 79, 81
stomachache 138
stomachache 138
stress reduction 13, 114, 122, 123, 124–5,
135, 141
stroke 137

T
tailbone reflex area
golf-ball sequence 106, 108
left hand sequences 74, 75, 94, 95
maps 16, 17
right hand sequence 81
techniques
desserts 60–5, 82–5
finger-walking 56–7
hook & back-up 58
rotating on a point 59
thumb-walking 54–5
warm-up/relaxation exercises 46–7,
143, 145, 149
teeth reflex area
left hand sequences 74, 75, 86, 94, 95
maps 18, 19
right hand sequences 80, 101
tendon glide exercises 46, 149
tendonitis 41
tension relief 130, 131, 139
testicle see ovary/testicle reflex area
thumb-walking 54–5
thumbs 38
golf-ball sequence 102, 103, 106
hand concerns 140, 142, 143, 144
left hand sequences 66–9, 74–5, 86–9,
94–5
right hand sequences 78–81, 98–101
thyroid gland reflex area
golf-ball sequence 102, 109

left hand sequences 66, 67, 86, 87
maps 16–19
right hand sequences 79, 99
tiredness 52, 134, 146–7
tools
self-help 23, 44–5, 50, 51, 53, 145, 147,
151
see also golf balls

U V W
upper back reflex area
golf-ball sequence 104, 105, 109
left hand self-help sequence 88, 89, 90,
91, 92, 93, 96, 97
left hand sequence 68, 69, 70, 71, 73,
76, 77
maps 16–19
right hand sequences 78, 79, 80, 81, 99,
100
urinary incontinence 136
uterus/prostate gland reflex area
children 111
left hand sequences 76, 77, 96, 97
maps 18, 19
menstrual cramps & PMS 139
right hand sequences 81, 101
vibrating wand 51, 147, 151
waistline, lateral marker 14, 15, 18, 19
walk-down/pull-against
arthritis 151
backache & neck pain 129
commuters 117
golf ball sequence 109
headaches 126, 127
insomnia 139
left hand sequences 66, 67, 75, 77, 86,
87
right hand sequences 78, 98, 99, 100,
109
techniques 64, 83
tired & sore hands 147
warm-up/relaxation exercises 43, 46–7, 49,
143, 144, 145
water intake 123
wax baths 53, 147, 151
webbing
left hand sequences 68–9, 70–1, 88–91
right hand sequences 78–81, 98–101
see also specific reflex areas located in
webbing (e.g. solar plexus)
work 140
see also keyboarding & office work

Z
zones & zone charts 11, 14–15

ACKNOWLEDGMENTS

Authors' acknowledgments

Our very special thanks to the editorial and design team for their exceptional work on this book. To photographer Ruth Jenkinson and her assistants Rupert Peace and Sarah Bailey; models Max Bollinger, Sarah Clive, Renato Defazio, Gemma Howarth, Luke Jenkinson, Gunilla Johansson, Sergio Marini, Roberto Peter, Sheila Power, Tonia and those little babies: Callie Cashmore-Bailey, David Moran-Cashmore, and Amelia Price.

And to the Dorling Kindersley team of Mary-Clare Jerram, Penny Warren, Marianne Markham, Shannon Beatty, Peggy Sadler, Irene Lyford, Toni Kay and her husband Richard Kay, who drew the arrows.

Publisher's acknowledgments

Dorling Kindersley would like to thank the following people for their help and participation in this project: Ruth Jenkinson and her assistants Rupert Peace and Sarah Bailey for photography; Max Bollinger, Callie Cashmore-Bailey, Sarah Clive, Renato Defazio, Gemma Howarth, Luke Jenkinson, Gunilla Johansson, Sergio Marini, David Moran-Cashmore, Roberto Peter, Sheila Power, Amelia Price and Tonia for modeling; Richard Kay for illustrations; Ann Baggaley for editorial assistance and Sue Bosanko for the index.

Dorling Kindersley would also like to thank HoMedics for the use of their ParaSpa™ Deluxe Paraffin Bath, which features on pages 53 and 147. Visit their website at www.homedics.co.uk

Picture credits

10–11: Ann Gillanders, The British School of Reflexology/ International Institute of Reflexology Picture researchers: Myriam Megharbi and Romaine Werblow.

The publisher would like to thank the following for their kind permission to reproduce their photograph on page 11: Ann Gillanders, The British School of Reflexology (www.foot.com)/ International Institute of Reflexology.